THE INJURY GUIDE

THE INJURY GUIDE

ELIMINATE PAIN, HEAL YOUR INJURIES, AND KEEP MOVING FOREVER

Dr. Erin Boynton MD

This book is written for informational purposes only. It is not intended as a diagnostic tool, prescription manual, or substitute for the advice and care of a qualified medical professional. Please consult with your doctor or other healthcare professional for recommendations that are specific to your health needs, before making any decisions that could affect your health. The publisher and authors of this book expressly disclaim to the fullest extent permitted by law any liability arising directly or indirectly from the use or misuse of the information contained herein.

PENGUIN
an imprint of Penguin Canada, a division of Penguin Random House Canada Limited

Canada • USA • UK • Ireland • Australia • New Zealand • India • South Africa • China

First published 2026

Penguin Canada
A division of Penguin Random House Canada
320 Front Street West, Suite 1400
Toronto, Ontario, M5V 3B6, Canada
penguinrandomhouse.ca

The authorized representative in the EU for product safety and compliance is Penguin Random House Ireland, Morrison Chambers, 32 Nassau Street, Dublin D02 YH68, Ireland, https://eu-contact.penguin.ie

LIBRARY AND ARCHIVES CANADA CATALOGUING IN PUBLICATION

Title: The injury guide : eliminate pain, heal your injuries, and keep moving forever / Erin Boynton MD.
Names: Boynton, Erin, author.
Description: Includes index.
Identifiers: Canadiana (print) 20250161753 | Canadiana (ebook) 20250168936 | ISBN 9780735247246 (softcover) | ISBN 9780735247253 (EPUB)
Subjects: LCSH: Pain—Treatment—Handbooks, manuals, etc. | LCSH: Wounds and injuries—Treatment—Handbooks, manuals, etc. | LCGFT: Handbooks and manuals.
Classification: LCC RB127 .B69 2026 | DDC 616/.0472—dc23

Cover design by Talia Abramson
Cover image: © martinussumbaji / Adobe Stock
Book design by Talia Abramson
Typeset by Terra Page

Printed in Malaysia

10 9 8 7 6 5 4 3 2 1

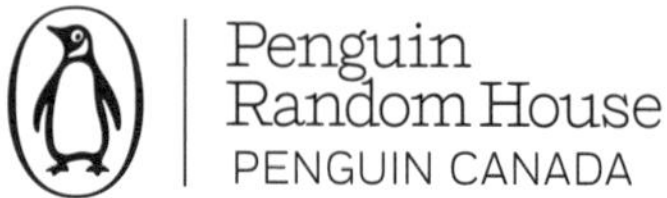

To all those who have gone on this movement journey with me.
Life is motion. Let's keep moving together!

CONTENTS

INTRODUCTION

A New Prescription for Pain

It was March 2003, and the New York Yankees were in town for the Toronto Blue Jays' home opener. A beautiful evening, the roof of the stadium was open, welcoming the fresh spring air. The smell of popcorn, vendors yelling "Ice-cold beer," and the crack of the bat heightened the excitement that the first day of baseball brings to our city. Thousands of vocal New York fans had travelled to Toronto to support their beloved Yankees, which added even more energy.

I was the orthopaedic surgeon for the Blue Jays, on call to manage any player injured on the field. Working with the Jays was very satisfying, and it was a hard-earned privilege to be the first woman to work as an orthopaedic surgeon in Major League Baseball. We had a lot of fun together too. I had earned the players' respect as I was able to communicate with them not only as a surgeon but as an elite athlete myself. I have always loved sport, and I know first-hand what it's like to suffer multiple wear and tear injuries. I've certainly had my share throughout my athletic career. Those experiences are what drew me to the orthopaedic profession and the subspecialty of sports medicine.

At that game, the team's physician, Dr. Ron Taylor, and I were discussing the fact that the medical malpractice insurance company we'd been using had recently decided it was no longer willing to cover professional sports physicians. Apparently, the risks were deemed too high. We were nervous that someone would get injured while we were sorting out our insurance issues. If we made a mistake and were sued, it could cost us our homes. Sure enough, just as we were hoping it would be a quiet evening, head trainer George Poulis came through loud and clear on my walkie-talkie: "Doc! We need you on the field—now!"

I ran down to the dugout and prepared to walk out to third base where New York's Derek Jeter was writhing in pain. Poulis met me and filled me in: Jeter had slid into third and hit his left shoulder on Jays catcher Ken Huckaby's knee, dislocating it.

When I got to third base, the Yankees trainer was trying to put the shoulder back in place. Jeter was in a lot of pain and as a result was resisting the help. His teammates helped us get Jeter into a golf cart and back to the training room. This was where I had to perform my magic.

Jeter was standing there, cradling his arm as if holding a baby, while Dr. Taylor and the Yankees trainer were sweating in the corner, wondering what I was going to do with their star player. "Bend over," I told Jeter in a very firm voice. As he did, I used gravity to relax the muscles and gently slid the bones back into place; he did not even know what happened. Immediately Jeter felt better. He moved his arm around in a circle and looked at me, amazed. "Thanks, doc! Can I go play?" The short answer to that was "No!"

After the fact, I learned that as I had approached Jeter at third base, a local radio announcer commented, "Oh look, there goes a woman to console Derek Jeter." When I started my career, only 2 percent of orthopaedic surgeons were women. I was told that I had to be twice as good as any male orthopaedic surgeon in order to keep my position with the team. Although I faced many challenges throughout my career, enough for a book all their own, these same experiences drove me to think differently and develop a special approach to wear and tear injury.

While acute traumatic injuries—like the one Derek Jeter experienced that day—often stick out in our minds, there's more to injuries and the pain that stems from them than what we experience in those extreme moments. Many people cannot, in fact, point to a specific event as the source of their pain or injury. There are the far more insidious injuries that develop slowly over time from, say, working on a factory line or lifting more weight than your body can handle. In time, the pain from these seemingly insignificant injuries becomes something you can't ignore.

This book is not about how to manage an acute shoulder dislocation, like Derek Jeter had. It's about how to turn back the hands of time—how to deal with wear and tear injuries so you don't have to live with chronic pain or give up all the activities you love to do. If you're thinking wear and tear injuries are just for "old" people, read on. Wear and tear can happen to anyone at any age, to anybody who does a repetitive motion or maintains one posture, like sitting. While I've always loved working with professional athletes, there's nothing more rewarding than giving regular people the ability to continue with their physical jobs, enjoy their gardens, or hit balls on the golf course.

In this book you will learn why a rotator cuff tears or a lumbar disc herniates and how arthritis develops in a knee. If you understand how your movement leads to wear and tear in your body, you can learn how to undo years of damage and prevent further degeneration by promoting a regenerative healing phase. From the tennis player with the sore shoulder whose serve is weakening to the parent with back pain who can no longer lift their children to the long-distance runner with painful knees to the office worker with a sore neck and all the other people who experience everyday pain that interferes with their ability to work, play, and have fun—this book is for you.

I have a unique approach to wear and tear injuries. I spent 16 years at university to hone my surgical craft. I was expertly trained to surgically repair ruptured tendons and torn ligaments and to replace arthritic joints. I loved the work. The surgical mentality is definitely "broken bone, fix it," and that clarity in approach was satisfying. However, early in my career, I noticed that surgical repairs fail after some time. I realized if I did not address *why* the body broke, then the repaired tissue would fail just like the original tissue had.

Years before I started treating pro baseball players, I had a mid-sized clinic at Toronto's Mount Sinai Hospital, where I worked as a sports doctor and surgeon. When you blew out your shoulder after throwing a vicious fastball or "did something weird" to your neck while working in the garden, I was the doctor you came to see. The problem was that was a lot of people.

Even with two secretaries, my office was a zoo. I saw 150 to 200 patients every week. The wait for a simple consultation was nine months. We had people phoning in every morning, desperate for a last-minute cancellation, and my assistant's inbox was overflowing with a never-ending river of requests and referrals. We could barely keep up.

By the time those patients walked through our clinic doors, they were usually desperate for help. Many had tried it all, from cortisone injections to physiotherapy sessions, with little to no improvement. Chronic pain kept them from sleeping properly, and injury kept them from doing the things they loved. Their lives were miserable. Worse still, if they needed surgery, they'd have to wait all over again, and this time it wouldn't be nine months—it would be two years.

Of course, I wanted to help each and every one of these patients. I knew what it was like to live with pain, but my hands were tied. There were just too many patients and not enough time. What I needed was a non-surgical solution. I needed something *new*.

So, I went ahead and booked my patients for surgery, but always with one major caveat: I didn't want them to rest while waiting. I wanted them to move. This advice was as surprising to them as it likely is to you. Rest, we're told, is the great panacea. It's the most commonly prescribed treatment in the world. But our bodies were made to move, and how we move determines how we heal.

So, I prescribed my patients exercises—ranging from complex isometric motions to simple stretches—and sent them on their way. It was not my surgical training that led me to this discovery but my life experience in sport. I had experimented with my own wear and tear injuries and learned what needed to change in how I moved my body. I shared these movement tips with my patients. They did their homework, sometimes with the aid of a physiotherapist and sometimes without, and then something special happened: They started to feel better. Much better. The same people who had cried in my office after learning there was a two-year wait for surgery would often come back at their three-month follow-up, saying they didn't need surgery at all. With the help of the exercises I prescribed, their injuries had resolved themselves. The exercises allowed the damaged tissues to heal by taking the pressure off the painful part of their body. All by changing how they moved.

Instead of dissecting the tissues, I dissected the issues. Why did the tendon tear or the disc herniate? What was it about my patient that caused their body to break down? I began to notice patterns: Soft tissues would become tight, which led to an imbalance in the body, which changed how the muscles worked. These compensations in movement were the body's attempt to protect itself, but eventually, when the body could not compensate any longer, tissues would tear, inflammation and pain would ensue, and function would be lost. I came to understand that most doctors and therapists were focused on treating what was broken or on decreasing inflammation, but they did not get to the root cause of why the body was breaking down. Certainly, their approach can help to temporarily decrease symptoms, but if you do not get to the root cause, the problem continues and progresses over time.

Think about a new car with a misaligned wheel. At first, the tire will tolerate the misalignment, but after miles of driving, you may notice that the tire is getting thin. If you stop driving, the tire stops wearing. Resting may prevent progression of the tire injury, but as soon as you start driving again, the wear and tear will progress, and eventually a hole will develop. If you take your car to the mechanic and they replace the tire, you will be fine for a while, but the wear and tear will start all over again. The mechanic must recognize that the tire needs to be realigned so the wear and tear stops. This is where I differ in my approach.

In this book, you will learn my approach to relaxing the tissues, correcting imbalances, and repatterning muscles to realign the musculoskeletal system—all of which allows your body to heal and stay active. This is not just a philosophy but a step-by-step approach based on science and clinical experience, not to mention my own experiences as an athlete. Like any strong structure, our body must have a foundation. I will teach you what comprises our Foundation for Movement: how to build your own foundation and how to keep it over your lifetime of activity. The single most common cause of wear and tear injuries is going through life without the proper Foundation for Movement. I want to empower you with this knowledge so you can stay active and pain free over your entire life.

Unfortunately, not all of us can avoid the knife. Sometimes surgery is necessary. But our bodies have an incredible capacity to remodel, and if we can harness that power through movement, most of our injuries will go away. And crucially, I've learned that if we don't determine why part of the musculoskeletal system broke down in the first place, the surgical repair will eventually fail in exactly the same manner. Even when surgery is necessary, using targeted movements to retrain how the body moves allows that part to heal and prevents further injury. No one wants to go through the same surgery twice.

This philosophy also applies well beyond surgery. How many times have you gone to your doctor in pain and they've given you some medication or, even worse, told you to stop doing what you love to do? Maybe you leave their office feeling better or even experiencing no pain at all, or perhaps you try some form of therapy, only to find your pain returns when you return to your activities. Your family doctor refers you to a surgeon, who maybe tells you that you're *heading* for a joint replacement or an operation to fix your torn tendon, meniscus tear, or arthritic back, but that your condition is not bad enough to warrant surgery. Yet you still have pain and can't resume your active life.

No one wants to stop doing the things they love, and no one wants to be limited in their day-to-day life. With this book, you will learn to manage pain, heal your injuries, and keep moving forever. Plain and simple. You'll learn how the way you've moved throughout your life thus far has led to parts of your body breaking down. You'll understand how movement affects your herniated disc, your arthritic knee, your inflamed rotator cuff—whatever it is—and you can take control of your own healing so that your body can recover and regenerate. You may even be able to avoid that surgery. But if you can't, you'll want to protect yourself so you don't wear the new part out again. The key is to learn how to establish and maintain a foundation for pain-free movement.

First, you will learn the fundamentals of pain. Pain is the body's voice, and I will share with you how to listen to this voice and understand its language. The body's voice is key in guiding how you move. Then I will discuss how our muscles, tendons, and joints break down, because once you understand this, you can put them back together again. You will learn the most common reasons that the body breaks down as well as an approach to movement that uses scientific principles to heal yourself.

Movement really is medicine, and I want to empower you to heal yourself using movement. The best way to do this is by teaching you how to keep moving despite wear and tear injuries. I have seen the body from both the inside and out, and I want to share my understanding of how you can work with your wear and tear injuries to restore your Foundation for Movement—the fundamental base of support that allows effective movement—in the best way possible. When it comes to healing the body with movement, we will focus on the five most common areas of our foundation that fall apart, and I'll offer movement solutions to restore that fundamental base of support. Not only will you learn how to assess your foundation, but you will also learn how to fix any deficiencies you discover through exercise. Learning how to keep moving safely whether you're in pain or not will allow you to live an active pain-free life.

PART I

Understanding Your Body and the Effects of Wear and Tear

CHAPTER 1

Your Body and the Gift of Movement

Life is motion. Movement shapes us in so many ways. Some movements are beneficial and can improve health, generally. But when and how we move can also lead to degeneration of our body. The most important gift we have is our mobility. Once it stops, or our movements become too repetitive, problems begin. Before we learn how to move better, we need to understand our body and what makes it so special.

If I could give you some advice: Resist skipping ahead to find the treatment plan particular to your condition. I know it's tempting, especially if you're hurting and desperate for a solution. These basics are here for a reason: to give you the necessary tools to understand and transform your body, and as you'll soon see, a big part of the power to heal your own body comes from being able to see the bigger picture.

Everything Is Interconnected

Even when you think you're only moving one part of your body, the reality is that movement at one joint can affect or produce movement at others. We often refer to this as the kinetic chain. Imagine Serena Williams as she prepares to hit with her forehand. As the ball sails over the net, she runs into position and prepares her body, bending and coiling as she brings back her racquet. Then as the ball gets closer, she uncoils, springing up, transferring the kinetic energy—the energy of a body in motion—from her legs, hips, and core through her arm, unleashing a blistering forehand. The strength of her forehand isn't in her arm; it's the combination of her legs, core, and arm all working in tandem, the transfer of kinetic energy through each link in the chain. And while the kinetic chain is vital to great performance, it's equally important in safeguarding against injury.

The longer I work as an orthopaedic surgeon, and the more I am involved with functional movement, the more relevant this concept becomes. I no longer look at a muscle, bone, or joint in isolation. We need to understand how all the parts come together to form a whole. As a surgeon, I was trained to look at the one specific part of the system that had broken down, but now I understand that the broken piece must be viewed in the context of the whole body.

There are key players in our body's movement system that everyone should know about. Understanding how they are all connected is our starting point for lifelong pain-free movement.

Fascia: The Key to Our Connectedness

Our body is not comprised of many separate pieces that come together to form a whole. It's better to think of it as one system that has many parts, and the key to this interconnectedness is a tissue known as fascia.

Fascia is more than just a type of tissue, though. It is its very own network, an intricate web of connective tissue that weaves through and envelops every part of your body, from the biggest bone down to the tiniest nerve ending, connecting every cell. You might think of the fascial network as a kind of biological glue, holding all of your body's bits in place. It is also a major conductor of nerve impulses, transmitting information about how much tension is in the tissue and where our body is positioned in space.

Although the fascia is one large network, its component parts—which include the perimysium (connective tissue surrounding muscles), tendons, ligaments, joint capsules, and periosteum (fascial membrane coating a bone)—differ widely in size, density, and function. It can be confusing because much of our knowledge has focused on the separate pieces of the body, and we often describe a muscle, a bone, or a joint structure as a separate entity. But this tissue does not exist in isolation; it is part of the whole connective tissue network or the fascial system. The composition of different parts depends on the functional requirements, as well as on how the tissue is stressed. It is a two-way street. For instance, the fascia interwoven between muscle fibres is very thin and delicate, like the strands of a spiderweb, to allow for greater motion. The large fascial sheets along the back, however, are thick and dense, like leather; they're much less malleable but are great at absorbing heavy mechanical stress, such as the kind of stress your back might experience when lifting a heavy box.

Imagine the inside of an orange. The orange segments are surrounded by the exterior skin, and underneath is a thicker white pith that surrounds the entire orange and thins out between and within the sections of the orange itself. All of the orange is connected with no beginning or end. Our musculoskeletal system is connected in exactly the same way from the tip of the toes to the tip of the nose.

Until recently, we've understood the musculoskeletal system as 206 bones under all the muscles, surrounding the internal organs, and covered with skin. Now we view the body as a fascial template, created before we're even born, which outlines the shape of our body: one fascia with 600 muscle pockets. In the past, fascia concerned doctors only when it became a problem, like when the fascia in a runner's foot became inflamed after a marathon (plantar fasciitis). Until recently, medical students cutting open cadavers would toss out the fascia to get to what we thought really mattered: the bones, muscles, and vital organs. Fortunately, we now know better.

As a network, the fascia is also the body's largest sensory organ, and its function is to inform the brain about where the body is positioned in space. It works like this: Any time you move—say, to reach for a glass or kick a ball—your fascial network sends signals to your brain and spinal cord detailing what's happening and where the various parts of your body are located in space. Using this knowledge, the brain then makes adjustments as necessary, activating certain muscles, deactivating others, and so on. If you reach too far into the back seat of your car to grab your briefcase, and the fascia is stretched to its max, it will alert the brain, triggering a sensation to stop you from hyperextending your arm and damaging your shoulder. The further you hyperextend your arm, the more intense and painful the sensation will become.

Every time we move, our fascia and nervous system scramble to restore equilibrium. Remember snow globes from childhood? The peaceful scene in the globe becomes chaotic with one shake, with snow flying everywhere, until all the snow quietly settles and balance is restored. Well, every time you move a millimetre, there is a degree of "snow flying" in our bodies. The cells in our fascia sense this movement and work to restore peace and quiet, a new equilibrium with each new position.

Responding to mechanical stimuli is the very work that keeps us active and alive, enabling our body to remodel. Imagine an astronaut in space, floating in zero gravity for days on end. Without the force of gravity, there are fewer mechanical stimuli, and the fascia, muscles, and bones atrophy in response. Interesting studies are being conducted in space to understand the mechanisms of tissue loss and how we can apply those learnings to various disease states here on Earth. And that is the danger of not moving here on Earth: Whether it's lying in bed for days or sitting in one position for hours at the office, we need to move, at least a little bit, to shake up our neuromuscular snow globes and keep our cells on their toes. If you don't use it, you lose it.

On the flip side, too much motion can also cause problems. Excess mechanical stress and stimulation leads to thickening, or hypertrophy, of the fascia. If there is a lot of mechanical loading of the tissues, the cells sense this and make more tissue to help distribute the load and strengthen the body. This is what happens with our muscles when we do weight training.

Most people, for example, have thicker fascia on the outside of their thighs, the fascia lata. Here the fascia helps to absorb the load on the outside of our legs, which allows the muscles to remain balanced. If the thick fascia was not there to absorb the forces of lateral movement, the muscles on the outside of the leg would have to do this job, which could create problems with alignment of the joints, eventually accelerating wear and tear. Interestingly, if we compare a horseback rider's legs to those of someone who does not ride, we may find that the rider has a structure similar to the fascia lata along the *inside* of their leg. This change in fascial structure is an adaptive response to the extra force placed on the inside of a rider's legs as they attempt to control their horse. In some instances, this can be a good thing—we want our legs to be protected, after all—but if the body creates too much fascial tissue, it can alter the entire alignment of the rider's leg, limiting mobility and leading to future imbalances and abnormal wear and tear.

Bones: More Than Just Our Shape

The 206 bones in the human body form the skeletal framework that allows us to move, but they are so much more than structural pieces of your body. Every bone's unique size and shape is a reflection of its function. For example, the tiny bones in your hands allow for very fine movement, like writing. The femur, your body's biggest and strongest bone, which runs from the hip to the knee, acts as an attachment point for big muscles, such as the quadriceps and hamstrings, that work together to move your legs.

And yet it's also a mistake to see our bones only as attachment points. Bones are more than inert structures that give shape to our fascial fabric. Like muscles and fasciae, they will waste away in the absence of movement. This matters to anyone who wants a healthy lifestyle, but it's especially important to those of us pushing 50. After the age of 20, your bone mass decreases 1 to 2 percent per year if you do not intervene to combat that bone loss. We can combat bone loss with diet and exercise—even jumping. Whether you're bouncing to your favourite tune or taking a little hop down the final couple stairs, every jump is a little jolt to your system. The body responds by constructing new bone along the lines of stress.

Joints: Where Life Happens

If life is motion and if we move at our joints, then joints give us our life. We have many different types of motion. Fine motor skills, such as threading a needle, and gross motor movements, such as raising your arm overhead, all happen because we have joints.

A joint is the spot where two bones meet. Most of them move, and some do not. We are going to focus on the ones that move because they are the major joints that become injured in our lifetime. There are two kinds of joints that move: hinge joints and ball and socket joints. Hinge joints, like your toes and elbows, function much like a door hinge. A door opens and closes, but it can't move in circles. Ball and socket joints, like your hips and shoulders, can move in multiple planes of motion, giving us much greater freedom of movement. Knowing what kind of joint each one is helps us understand how to move better.

To round out our movements, accessories like cartilage, joint capsules, tendons, ligaments, and muscles are a must. These components are not really distinct separate structures, but a part of the interconnected fascial system. Still, it's simpler to describe them separately to give us a fuller picture of what's happening in our bodies.

JOINT CARTILAGE

If you've ever eaten a chicken wing, you've seen joint cartilage: the smooth white tissue at the end of every bone. It's the slippery surface that allows our bones to glide with almost no friction. Without it, our bones would be like two blocks of concrete scraping against each other.

As we start to lose our articular (joint) cartilage, whether through disease or everyday wear and tear (a process called arthritis), our bones generate more and more friction, which can cause joint inflammation, swelling, and pain. Unfortunately, articular cartilage has no blood supply, so it can't regenerate like other parts of our connective tissue. This is why we have to be especially careful to keep our articular cartilage safe.

JOINT CAPSULES

As the name suggests, joint capsules enclose and contain the joints. Each capsule has a lining rich with molecules that help lubricate the joint and provide nutrition to the articular cartilage. Because cartilage does not have a blood supply, it is very much in need of this external nutrition source. Joint capsules also act as stabilizers by limiting our movements so we don't dislocate our joints.

The structure and composition of joint capsules vary in type and complexity depending on the joint. Your finger, for instance, has a very simple joint capsule because a finger only needs to bend and extend. However, the joint capsule of the shoulder, which has a greater range of motion than any other joint in the body, is far more complicated. When your arm is at your side, the joint capsule in the shoulder is loose and baggy, like a shirt sleeve. But when you raise your arm, the capsule stretches and tightens. Without that extra tissue, you wouldn't have nearly as wide a range of motion.

Tendons and Ligaments

Tendons are strong flexible cords that attach muscle to bone. When a muscle contracts, it applies force to the attached tendon, causing the bone to move. That's why when a tendon is torn or injured, it's very hard to move certain parts of your body. A tendon's size and shape vary, depending on the function of the muscle to which it's attached. For instance, the tendons in your fingers are long and cylindrical with a great excursion (path of movement), enabling your tendons to cross over the myriad joints in your hand—like the knuckles, which allow your fingers a wide range of motion, including the ability to extend outward and close into a fist. The broad flat tendon in your rotator cuff, however, has a very small excursion, because unlike the tendons in your fingers, it moves within a very limited range and crosses over only a single joint. Its job is simply to keep the ball of the shoulder properly aligned in its socket when the shoulder moves. And as you might've already guessed, the muscles and tendons that cross more than one single joint tend to be most vulnerable to injury.

A partial injury to the tendon and the muscle to which it connects is called a *strain*. There are different degrees of strain depending upon how much tissue is damaged and range from minor partial injury to moderate partial injury to complete tearing of the structure. You may have heard someone tell you that they *sprained* their knee or their shoulder. The difference is that a sprain affects a ligament and not a tendon or muscle.

Ligaments are sturdy bands of tissue that connect bone to bone along the two sides of a joint, acting as guide wires to keep your joints and bones in proper alignment. Without ligaments, we'd have nothing to stop us from moving our arms and legs too far. We'd be constantly dislocating our shoulders, elbows, and knees.

Joint stability depends on more than just ligaments. It is determined by the joint capsule, the shape of the bone, and special structures such as the meniscus—a thin fibrous cartilage between the surfaces of some joints—all of which are fixed, or static, structures. Joint stability also relies on proprioception, the sensory feedback sent through our nervous system to our muscles, telling us where our body is positioned in space. So, when you move your arm or leg and there is excessive stretch on the proprioceptors, they signal the muscles to contract so that the joint doesn't dislocate. The small muscles surrounding a joint also play an important role in stability by contracting and helping to keep a joint aligned. This is known as dynamic stability, and it's especially important if you have lax ligaments to begin with or you have torn a ligament.

There is a spectrum of instability from partial loss of alignment, referred to as a subluxation, to a complete loss of normal alignment, a dislocation. What's the big deal if you have joint instability? The first—and most obvious—is pain. Dislocations hurt. And they can be dangerous. One patient of mine dislocated his shoulder delivering a calf. Another did it while scuba diving when he caught his suit on a rock; he almost drowned. But even if your dislocation isn't deadly, it can still cause damage.

Each time the joint dislocates, it can damage the joint surface or accessory structures like the meniscus. Interestingly, patients with atraumatic instability tolerate dislocation with far less joint damage than those with traumatic instability. This may have to do with the forces required to cause the dislocation—more soft tissue damage occurs with the latter.

In addition to the functional short-term problems, you also have to worry about the long-term: namely, arthritis. Arthritis can be so severe that it causes permanent loss of motion with pain so bad you need a joint replacement. Whether you develop arthritis depends on a number of factors, but the more you dislocate a joint, the more likely it is.

Some ligaments are intra-articular (inside the joint), like the anterior cruciate ligament (ACL); others are extra-articular (outside the joint), like the medial collateral ligament (MCL). Others are just a thickening of the joint capsule, like in the shoulder joint. Injuries happen when the ligament is torn from the bone or within the ligament itself (a mid-substance tear). There is a spectrum of injury that ranges from an internal "stretch" of the ligament to a partial tear to the worst—a complete tear of the ligament structure. Treatment for these injuries depends on particulars: the joint, the location, the specific ligament involved, and the types of activities you participate in.

Muscles

Muscles are the main engine for our bodies. When they work, we move. In our bodies, we have both involuntary muscles and voluntary muscles. Involuntary muscles work in the background without any effort from you. Your heart is a muscle, and right now, it is beating on its own. It's the same for the muscles in your intestines, which don't require any kind of conscious activation. Are they important? Absolutely. But you're not exactly at risk of straining your intestinal muscles during a game of ultimate frisbee.

Voluntary muscles are the ones you *do* have to consciously contract and relax, like your biceps and hamstrings. They're what enable bodily motion so we can run, jump, and swing a baseball bat. Our muscles are pressure pumps, creating waves of stress that flow through our kinetic chain to cause motion. These voluntary muscles create movement by applying force to the fascial system, most specifically tendons, which in turn cause the bones to move. Muscles are a critical piece of our puzzle because they are the one tissue that we can focus on to control the entire musculoskeletal system. When a muscle contracts, it not only tells the body how to move; it also tells the cells in the fascia that surrounds it, and is intertwined with it, what to do. The way we move, or contract, our muscles controls how pressure flows through our body, which is the critical factor in how we either heal or break down.

So how do our muscles work together to produce movement? Our 600 or so muscles each have a specific job to do, which allows for efficient motion. If all of them contracted at the same time, we would not move! The muscles work together like an orchestra: Some play loudly, others softly; they have to come into the song at the right time; and they have to be in the right key (tight or loose enough). Our brain and our fascial system are the conductor, while the muscles, bones, and joints are the various instruments.

THE THREE TYPES OF MUSCLE CONTRACTIONS

CONCENTRIC: The muscle contracts and shortens. When you lift a bag of groceries by bringing your wrist toward your shoulder, the biceps muscle contracts and shortens.

ECCENTRIC: The muscle contracts and lengthens. When you lower a bag of groceries until your arm is fully extended, the biceps muscle contracts and lengthens.

ISOMETRIC: The muscle is engaged and contracted, but the joint angle does not change. When you hold a bag of groceries steady with your elbow bent at a 90-degree angle, your biceps muscle engages and contracts and the elbow doesn't move.

Some of the joints in our body are more mobile, while others are more stable in their movements. Toes, for example, are mobile, while the midfoot is stable. Ankles are mobile, and knees are stable. Hips are mobile, while your core is stable, and so on. Our body is designed so that the joints located beside one another have opposite functions. This allows coordinated movement and is essential to a properly functioning kinetic chain. When you bend down to pick up your shoes from the floor, the joints work together, with the toes mobile and midfoot stable, ankle mobile and knee stable, hip mobile and core stable, and so on. If the ankle or the hip have lost mobility, then we have to compensate somewhere along the kinetic chain in order to pick up the shoe; often our knees or our back have to move more than they are normally expected to. When we have compensations, we do not transfer the mechanical stress through the kinetic chain smoothly. Imagine that wave of pressure being stopped at a dam, and all of the force being applied to one area of the body. We can get away with this once in a while, but if it goes on for years, our body will begin to break down.

One section of the orchestra is called the prime movers, and they include almost all the muscles you're likely familiar with: the quadriceps, triceps, and calves, among others. Their job, as the name suggests, is to initiate movement. When we want to bend our arm, the muscles on the front of the arm contract while the muscles on the back must relax, or else motion would not occur. Some muscles cross two joints, so when they contract, they will potentially move both joints. For example, the biceps brachii (often just called the biceps) crosses both the elbow and the shoulder. We need an internal stabilizing force to prevent the shoulder from moving when you are trying to bend your elbow so you can move your hand toward your mouth. If your shoulder could not stay stable, then contracting the biceps would move both the elbow and shoulder and you couldn't get your hand to your mouth. If the prime movers and stabilizers do not work in concert, then the movement song is out of key and chaotic. But when the muscles in the core and shoulder contract to hold the shoulder in the correct position, the elbow can bend properly. It is important that the joint above and below the one that is moving are stabilized.

It's not necessarily important for you to be able to distinguish between different functions of the muscles or joints in the body, but it is useful to know how changes in one joint can affect another. If a joint that's supposed to be mobile stiffens, it will have an impact on the joints above and below; the converse is also true. Maintaining your joints' flexibility and stability is key to normal movement. When a joint loses either mobility or stability, our system has to compensate for this loss in order to function.

Remember the alternating pattern in our joint system: one joint's job is primarily to move, while the next joint must stabilize the segment. When our neuromuscular orchestra listens to the conductor and everyone does their job, movement is effortless. Unfortunately, some tissues get out of key, some play too softly or too loudly or, even worse, forget to play at all. When this happens and another tissue steps in, we call it a compensation.

When one muscle does the job of ten, problems develop. Nobody likes to do more than their fair share or do a job that they were not meant to do. Compensations often occur at the muscular level. Sometimes muscles do not activate and contract when they are supposed to; as a result, another muscle must pitch in. We see this most commonly with the deep core stabilizing muscles, particularly if we sit or stand with bad posture. The bad posture causes the stabilizing muscles to be too long or too short, and muscles don't like that, so they shut off and go to sleep. When this happens, the nervous system automatically recruits another muscle, usually one of the prime movers, to take over and get the job done. These muscle compensations are extremely common and wreak havoc by creating imbalances in the musculoskeletal system.

Anyone out there have tight hamstrings? Do you stretch every day, working hard to get those hammies to lengthen, only to find that an hour after you stretched, they are short and tight again? This is a common compensation. The usual job of the hamstrings, which cross both the hip and the knee, is more of a stabilizing function at the hip, but if the glutes shut down because we sit on them for 8 to 12 hours a day, then the hamstrings have to compensate and perform hip extension. Hip extension is not really what the hamstrings are designed to do most of the time, so the muscles rebel and get tight and sometimes painful, complaining because the hamstrings are doing the job of something else.

Another common compensation happens with our foot and ankle from wearing shoes all day long. Our feet are crucial components of the kinetic chain. They are usually the first contact with the ground and therefore an important starting point for good balance and a solid foundation. Shoes cause the intrinsic muscles of our feet to shut off. When this happens, tissues like the plantar fascia and the Achilles tendon must bear the extra stress, eventually wearing out and becoming painful. As you will soon learn, the solution here is not to treat only the overloaded hamstring, plantar fascia, or Achilles tendon. If you do not get to the real reason that these tissues are breaking down—that is, the compensations—you will never get better. For long-term improvement, you must fix the root cause of the issue, which is the movement compensation. Reactivating the glutes will allow the hamstrings to do their usual job and relax. Turning on the muscles in your feet will take the load off the plantar fascia and the Achilles, allowing them to repair.

HAVE YOU EVER HEARD OF THE "FOOT CORE"?

Approximately 19 small intrinsic muscles on the bottom of our feet are responsible for moving our toes and anchoring our feet to the ground by creating our normal arches. Together, they are the foot core. See if you can turn them on.

Place your bare foot on the ground, imagine a line from your first to fifth toe travelling along the ball of your foot, then imagine two lines, one going from the fifth and one from the first toe to the base of your fifth metatarsal (a bump halfway along your foot on the outside). Can you visualize that triangle? Gently spread your toes and apply even pressure across the ball of your foot, with very little weight in your heel. Now see if you can pull the base of the triangle toward the tip. That is how the muscles can create an arch.

As important as creating that arch is, these little muscles pull on the posterior fascial chain, which travels, you guessed it, along the back of our bodies from the tip of the toes to the tip of the nose! The muscular pull generates tension along the fascia, storing free energy and ensuring that other muscles along the posterior chain are at the optimal length to fire up. Here's a neat little neurological fact: The nerve roots that supply our gluteal muscles, our pelvic floor muscles, and our intrinsic foot muscles are the same. By contracting the foot intrinsics, you give a little boost to the pelvic floor and glutes, seriously enhancing your overall stability. When the right muscles are engaged, you feel light on your feet, stable, and balanced, and there's a great bounce in your step, as though you are walking on a mini trampoline.

For more complex motion, it is critical that we use our kinetic chain, engaging all parts of our musculoskeletal system to avoid injury. Remembering that muscles and fasciae are not separate entities, one of the critical actions of a muscle contraction is to produce tension along the whole body. These tissues are so interconnected that we commonly refer to them together as the myofascial system. Energy is stored in an elastic manner within the fascia; it is like preloading a spring. Ensuring that our movement orchestra is finely tuned, in key, performing at the right intensity, and in time will go a long way toward effortless movement because we'll be using our whole kinetic chain. Understanding what instruments in your orchestra are out of tune, imbalanced, or compensating will allow us to get to the root cause of the problem and improve the sound of your movement song.

In the next chapter, we will learn how to recognize when there's a problem, what those different problems may feel like, and how best to communicate that to a health care professional.

MOVEMENT MESSAGES

- You lose what you don't use. We are made to move, so use your musculoskeletal system every waking hour.
- We are connected from the tip of the toes to the tip of the nose. As we are one continuous interconnected system, movement in the toes can affect the hip or the arm or even the nose.
- Each segment of the musculoskeletal system has an individual function, either mobility or stability, yet everything must work together for optimal movement.
- Understanding how imbalances and compensations in the musculoskeletal system are the root causes of pain and movement dysfunction will open your eyes to the movement solutions.

CHAPTER 2

Pain Is the Body's Voice

Most of us think of pain as suffering, distress in its most raw and physical form. This is for good reason: Pain, whether from a scraped knee or a broken arm, is unpleasant. It hurts. But there is much more to pain.

Sometimes the source of pain is obvious, like in the examples mentioned above, but often it can be more difficult to locate. The uncertainty around pain, and when—if ever—it will subside, makes it feel like an invisible bogeyman hiding in our bodies, ready and waiting to do us harm.

What do we do when we feel pain? Naturally, we try to get rid of it. But if we look at pain objectively, we see that it isn't bad at all. Pain is our body's voice, alerting us to something we need to pay attention to.

If you swim underwater long enough, you'll feel pain in your lungs. That's your body telling you it needs oxygen. If you put your hand on a hot stove, you'll feel pain in your hand. That's your body telling you your skin is searing. If you don't eat anything all day, you'll feel a stomach pang. That's your body telling you it needs food. Pain is a message telling us something is wrong. If we listen to that message, we can fix the problem—you come up for air, you move your hand, or you eat something. But if we ignore the message, the problem gets worse. In some instances, if we ignore it long enough, the problem can progress to tissue breakdown and disease. Initially, pain is a signal that some action needs to be taken to restore balance to our system. Pain is a normal part of life and the body's only way to tell you that it needs something.

What do the pains in our muscles and joints mean? What is our body trying to tell us? In other words, what is "normal" pain and why does it happen? There are two major causes for musculoskeletal pain: either not enough fuel to run the body part, or too much mechanical load on the area. Let's imagine your body is a car. Both our bodies and our cars need fuel to keep moving. Our tissues need oxygen and chemical energy from food. When we are running low on energy supplies and our tank is almost empty, our muscles become painful. Let's call this metabolic pain. Have you ever run so far or fast that your leg muscles hurt? That pain is the cells in your muscles screaming that they need more oxygen or glucose in order to function. The body is telling you, *I am out of the things that I need to function, so time to stop and replenish.* Not enough fuel to sustain movement is one of the most common causes of pain in our connective tissues, especially muscles.

The second most common reason is mechanical. Remember the worn-out tire? If the wheels are out of alignment, then abnormal stress on the tire can eventually lead to a hole. Mechanical stress on our tissues (either too much compression or tension) can result in pain signals. This is that uncomfortable pulling sensation that you may have experienced across the front of your shoulder when you reach too far, or that tender feeling when someone gives you a bear hug. The message here is to remove the pressure before the tissue breaks down. This is an example of a normal way the body uses a pain signal to tell you that it needs something.

Our body's voice isn't always easy to understand. Even something as simple as a headache can have more than a dozen causes, from bad posture to severe arthritis. But if we can learn to listen to our pain, we'll become more attuned to what our body needs. It's human nature that we tend to ignore pain until we lose function. This is often when the pain has changed in character. No longer just a message that the body needs rebalancing, the pain has become associated with tissue damage (pathology). By better understanding our pain, we have a much better chance of preventing injuries from progressing to that point.

While there are many causes of physical pain, the focus of this book is wear and tear musculoskeletal injuries: pain in the fascial system, the muscles, tendons, bones, and joints. This is the pain you feel when you've pulled your back or injured your knee. And like all pain, musculoskeletal pain is a message, telling you that you're overusing or overloading a part of your body and, most importantly, that you have a problem in your

Foundation for Movement. In other words, imbalances and compensations are starting to throw off your fundamental base of support and interfere with effective movement.

Picture yourself in the grocery store. You thought it would be a short trip to pick up a couple of things, so you decided to forgo the cart. But now you're in line awkwardly cradling a dozen apples, three frozen pizzas, two avocados, and a bag of oats. As you wait for the gentleman in front of you to pay for his milk using change, your arms and back start to hurt. The longer he takes, the more the pain intensifies. You feel this pain because your muscles are being overworked. Thankfully, when you finally dump all of your groceries on the counter, the pain quickly dissipates.

The solution is not to stop buying groceries. Rather, a different grocery shopping strategy should be used. Instead of carrying everything at once, make two trips *or* strengthen your body to easily carry all those groceries. If you don't like either of these options, use a cart! The important thing here is that we must learn to listen to our bodies so that we know when they're being overloaded; we can then change our strategy to prevent pain and injury from happening in the first place.

Don't Kill the Messenger

Our first instinct when we feel pain is to quickly eliminate that distress. But sometimes it's easier or faster to ignore relatively minor pains. Some small pains go away on their own or are situation specific and don't require us to rethink how we do something. Problems arise when we do not listen to persistent pain and continue to act a certain way. Eventually our body will break down, and that is when the nature of pain changes. Pain is no longer warning us of a potential problem; pain is there because there is a problem. The trick is to learn to listen to your pain and take action before structural injuries take place.

It's natural to want to eliminate pain, but remember that pain is just information, telling us something needs our attention. There's a difference between out of balance and broken; we need to know how to gauge the pain we feel, so we can respond appropriately. There's a simple way to practise listening to your pain.

Are you in pain now? On a scale from 0 to 10, with 0 being no pain at all and 10 being the most severe pain, give your pain a rating. This is known as the numeric pain rating scale (NPRS), and it's a powerful tool we use to track the progress of our interventions as well as to nip problems in the bud before they progress too far. A score of 0–3 represents mild pain, 4–6 moderate pain, and 7–10 severe pain. Rate your pain regularly and observe trends over time.

We'll be using the NPRS later as a part of your history and assessment and to monitor your response to the program. Remember: Pain is a normal part of life, a protector that can tell us when something is out of balance. But pain can also alert us to a problem, telling us when tissue is actually damaged. Rating the severity of pain is a good first step, but it doesn't tell us everything we need to know. The language of pain can help us better understand when pain is protective or pointing to pathology.

By learning the vocabulary of pain, you will know how to describe what you feel to a doctor in a way they can easily decipher. No one can feel our pain for us, and it can be a tricky thing to describe to someone else. Understanding the most common types of pain, and the most common terms for them, helps us more quickly and more accurately find the source of the problem.

GENERAL MUSCLE SORENESS

If you've ever hit the gym really hard, you've probably suffered a workout hangover. Delayed-onset muscle soreness, or DOMS if you want to impress your gym-rat friends, is the muscular pain, stiffness, and soreness you feel 24 to 48 hours after you've worked them.

While DOMS can be painful, it does not last forever—it's just a bunch of muscular micro-injuries that, given time, will repair themselves and make you stronger. (That being said, I don't recommend regularly pushing yourself to such extremes that climbing the stairs after each workout feels like ascending Everest.) DOMS typically feels like a general soreness through the entire muscle. You often only notice sore muscles when you activate or poke them, and the soreness usually diminishes after two to three days, unless you went beast mode working on the house or on an all-day bike ride after a long layoff. Severe DOMS can largely be avoided by easing into more rigorous activities, which we'll discuss later.

People often wonder about continuing their workouts when they have DOMS. Unless your pain is so severe that you can't move at all, keep moving. You may need to decrease the intensity of your movement when you're experiencing DOMS, but doing something that allows your body and your muscles to be used, not abused, is actually good for recovery. Most people feel better after they go for a walk, swim, or ride a bike to get the motor running. This is called active recovery. Low-intensity movement will bring in a good blood supply to flush out the waste products of the extra-hard workout and deliver repairing molecules to speed up muscle regeneration. You can use the NPRS here to monitor your response to active rest. Once your pain is mild (0–3), you can resume your normal level of activity after a good warm-up. (Just don't overdo it.)

AN UNUSUAL CASE OF DOMS

Whiplash is the source of a lot of pain—and a lot of lawsuits. But what exactly causes whiplash? Well, think about what happens to your body during a car crash. The seat belt restrains your torso, but your head and neck continue moving forward at a violent speed, then jerk back at the moment of impact. To prevent catastrophic injury, the muscles in the neck and trapezius use everything they've got to slow and stabilize your head and neck. This can save your life, but it also comes at a cost: 24 to 48 hours later, your neck and shoulders will be almost unbearably stiff. Does that timeline seem familiar? It should, because whiplash is usually just a severe case of DOMS.

It's also possible that you've broken a bone or suffered some other traumatic injury, especially if the crash was bad. Before you do any exercising, get a doctor to examine you.

Once your doctor has given you the all clear, check out the Head, Neck, and Upper Back Routine in Chapter 5. Following these guidelines won't prevent all the pain and stiffness, but it will prevent a lot of it. And instead of it taking you two to three months to recover, it should take only a week or two.

BURNING MUSCLES

We know that DOMS is a normal consequence of pushing our muscles to the limit, but what about the pain you feel *while* you're exerting yourself?

Let's say you're on a family vacation to New York, climbing the stairs at the Statue of Liberty. As you hit the 150th step, a slow burn creeps into your hamstrings and quads. What is this pain trying to tell you? In this case, your muscles are shouting that they have no more fuel: *We need oxygen! We need glucose!* While uncomfortable, it's a perfectly normal sign that your muscles need something. The burning feeling in your muscles when you're active is what most people call "lactic acid," and it's transient. In truth, scientists have never been able to pinpoint exactly what causes this pain. It is thought, however, to be due to a combination of factors: micro-injuries, inflammation, and chemical and hormonal changes, including lactic acid. One thing we do know for sure is it will go away once you decrease the intensity of your activity or take a rest. Just Google "Sian Welch crawling to Ironman finish" to see the dramatic effects of your body running out of gas. A burning sensation is your body's way of telling you that the muscle is out of fuel and will stop doing its job (or fail) very soon.

TIGHT MUSCLES

Another common pain sensation you might feel occurs when you reach the end range of joint motion. Have you ever played crack the whip? You know, the game we played as kids. A group of us would hold hands, one end was the head, the other the tail. We would run or skate furiously in one direction until the leader suddenly changed direction. If you were at the end of the whip, you might feel your muscles stretching across the front of your chest as your arm was pulled behind your body, and that could become painful if you were to keep going. This is your body warning you that you have gone far enough, and hopefully you let go of your friend's hand. The farther your arm is pulled behind you, the more the tension grows, as does the tightness. If you push your range of motion beyond the point of this pain, you may tear the fascia, a ligament, a tendon, or a joint capsule. This is an example of how a pain signal protects us from moving too far and damaging our bodies. So be sure to let go before it is too late!

The tightness caused from overreaching is different from the feeling of tightness we experience when a muscle is too short and tight, a common example being our hamstrings. Many people have tight and painful hamstrings as a result of overuse. Why is this? When you sit at your desk all day long, your glutes (a.k.a. butt muscles) forget how to work—something called gluteal amnesia—so when it's time to stand up, our bodies compensate by using the hammies instead. When a muscle, the hamstring in this case, does a job that it's not meant to do, it can become short and tight as a result of being chronically overworked.

Your hamstrings could also be tight because of poor posture that leads to changes in the nervous system and what we call neuromuscular facilitation. If all the muscles in our body were to suddenly relax, we would topple over. This freaks our brain out. Of course, the hamstrings are working when we walk normally, but they should not be overworking. Say you are walking on an unstable surface, such as sand on a beach; if our brains perceive that we're going to lose our balance, then additional muscles are called into action so that we don't fall over. To maintain good posture, which is reflected in normal alignment and stability of our joints, our nervous system sends signals to always keep some muscles active, as a protective mechanism.

Whether your tightness is a result of overuse or neuromuscular facilitation, the key is to make sure the right muscles are doing their jobs: being active, alert, and functional when they're supposed to be.

We cannot forget stress as a trigger for tight muscles. If we have something going on in our lives that is taxing, it creates a feeling that we are not safe. Chronic stress increases the overall nervous energy in our body, which puts us in fight-or-flight mode. Our muscles, often those around our neck, respond by tightening up to be ready for action.

The pain or discomfort associated with muscle tightness is a message that needs to be listened to. If an affected muscle has a normal range of motion, then the signal most likely means you have reached the end of your range. If, however, your range of motion is limited, then you will have to investigate further. Is the loss of mobility due to a problem within the joint itself, or has there been shortening of the muscle due to injury or disuse? The pain that comes with a limited range of motion, while frustrating, is not something that should frighten you. Your body just needs attention. I will teach you how to address tight muscles later on.

TRIGGER POINTS IN MUSCLES

Trigger points, or "knots," often occur when one muscle is compensating for another. Unlike other kinds of muscle pain, which run through the entire muscle, the soreness of a knot will be contained to a smaller (pointed) area at the site of the knot. This pain caused by a trigger point is typically pretty steady throughout the day, whether you're using the muscle or not. Sometimes the pain will radiate into another part of your body and be associated with a diffuse tingling or burning feeling elsewhere. You might be nervous that you have a pinched nerve, but it's important to remember that the referred tingling associated with a trigger point can affect a broad area.

The solution is to address the compensation or dysfunction. For a bit of relief in the short term, you can try a massage or active self-myofascial release (ASMR), which involves gently massaging the affected area yourself and pairing the massage with movement. Later, you'll learn how to use this technique to get to the root cause of muscle knots so you can prevent them from coming back.

MUSCLE SPASMS AND CRAMPING

A little different than overworked muscles, muscle spasms happen involuntarily in response to an acute injury. There's no actual problem with the muscle in spasm—it is responding in a protective manner so that no more damage can occur. Say you injure one of the little joints in your back or neck (facet joints). The surrounding muscles will automatically contract and stay contracted until the acute injury resolves. This is because the body is trying to protect the area. With the muscle going into spasm, there can be no motion of the affected joint, and that allows the damaged area to heal. Releasing the spasm in a muscle is fine, but you have to make sure that other muscles in the area are awake and ready to work. When all the muscles that are supposed to be supporting a joint are awake and engaged, they will help off-load the injured area, and inflammation and pain will decrease.

Cramping is a little different from a spasm, although both can be extremely painful. Generally, a cramp happens when a muscle has been completely depleted of fuel; it is exhausted. Cramping is commonly associated with dehydration. Have you ever awoken in the middle of the night with a severe cramp in your gastroc (calf muscle)? I have been more than rudely awakened in the middle of the night with a severe pain in my calf and my toe pointing at an extreme. What you have to do is grab your foot and ankle and dorsiflex the ankle (close the angle in the front), which will cause a reciprocal inhibition in the calf muscle (more on this term later). Cramping may also be associated with a tendon or muscle injury. The body's voice is loudly telling you to rest and give your muscle some food or drink. A slightly different cramp can occur when you first start to awaken a muscle that has not been working properly for a while. As you attempt to contract the muscle, you can go from nothing (relaxed muscle) to maximal contraction too quickly, and our nervous system gets carried away. This is actually a good sign because a muscle that cramps, in this situation, is a muscle that can be strengthened. Just move into the contraction more slowly, ramping the intensity gradually to your maximum. After a severe muscle cramp, you may experience DOMS for 24 hours or so; don't be alarmed.

POINTED BURNING OR TINGLING

Generally, this pain is the result of a nerve being stretched or pinched. If you feel this during activity, back off and continue within a range of motion that doesn't cause it. One of the most common causes is from sitting at your desk. If you lean on bent elbows for hours at a time, looking at the computer screen, or talking on the phone, the ulnar nerve, which is on the inside of the joint, can be squished. You may experience numbness and tingling in your baby and ring fingers. As soon as you straighten your elbow, voila, the numbness resolves. Burning and tingling caused by nerve impingement has much more localized symptoms than burning and tingling caused by a trigger point, which can affect the whole arm or leg.

PINS AND NEEDLES

This is the feeling of blood returning to an extremity after it's been blocked for a period of time. This would happen to me when I'd fall into a deep sleep after being on call for 36 hours. Often I would sleep on my arm, and when I woke up, my arm would be "full of pins and needles." I remember one morning when my alarm went off, I couldn't control my numb arm and hit myself in the face. I thought someone was attacking me! With one change in position so the blood can return, this sensation quickly resolves.

SHARP JOINT PAIN

If you feel sharp pain during movement, you should stop, because it indicates the possible pinching or tearing of one of the joint's connective tissues. If you feel this, you need to avoid the sharp pain as much as possible. In many cases, lifelong repetitive movements will cause an imbalance in how one of the connective joint tissues is being loaded. When it's loaded in a bad way, it becomes painful.

The way to get things working right will be different for every case, but it likely includes addressing tissue restrictions and ensuring that muscles are active and strong and that movement patterns are clean. I will teach you how to correct the imbalance and change how you move so that the tissue can heal or at least stop deteriorating.

ACHY JOINTS

If your joints are achy throughout the day, it's likely that they are degenerating and are inflamed as a result. If your aching is chronic, it is usually called osteoarthritis. To stop the progression of chronic osteoarthritis, it's important to look at the big picture of your physical health, including daily activity, exercise, nutrition, sleep, stress, and any prescription medications.

If an achy joint comes and goes, it could be the result of a high volume of loading on the joint. For example, I get achy knees when I play in a tennis tournament. The matches are intense, and in the back of my mind, I still think I can make it on the WTA Tour.

Whether chronic or not, to settle down pain and prevent swelling, you can try contrast showers: alternating 30 seconds of hot and then cold water on the area three to five times. This will provide temporary relief while you work on your Foundation for Movement.

Even if you have chronic pain due to a degenerative condition, you can benefit from looking at your Foundation for Movement and making corrections to halt the progression of your issues. It may even be possible to reverse the damage that has been done. On a foundational level, I will teach you how to correct your movement patterns and unload the painful joint. Changing how you move, not stopping movement, is key.

GOOD PAIN VERSUS BAD PAIN

Injuries have other telltale signs, like swelling and the inability to maintain your form or posture. That said, if you've really done something serious to a muscle, tendon, bone, or ligament, you'll know it. Even when sudden sharp pain isn't indicative of a serious injury, it is, at the very least, a message from your body worth listening to. So, if you feel this, stop and consider the cause. Is your form bad? Are you lifting too much weight? Did you not warm up properly? Go slow and take the time to figure it out. Your body will thank you for it. And if you develop swelling, loss of joint motion, or weakness, contact a doctor.

It's important to listen to the various painful sensations you experience to learn how your body speaks. With attention, you will be able to discern when pain is just a sign that you have worked hard in the gym or stretched your body far enough, and when pain signals tissue damage. Understanding the relationships between activity and pain, and specifically how you were moving or not moving, can give you valuable information for the future. Every time you experience pain, it is an opportunity to learn more about your body—your house—and what you can do to make your house a home.

The Emotions of Pain

Pain can be emotional and pain can be physical, and the line between the two isn't always clear. The death of a close friend can hurt just as much as any physical wound. And when we're facing a breakup, there's a reason we describe our heart as broken. We feel emotional pain in our bodies. Sadness, jealousy, and anger—these things hurt.

The way we react to pain can have as much influence on how we feel as the injury itself. Negative emotions directed toward an injury can intensify physical pain, and positive ones can alleviate it. It's easier said than done, but the better we're able to manage our emotional response to pain, the better we're able to manage pain itself.

Let's say you cut your finger. When you do, the cut creates a signal that goes from your finger to your brain that says, *Ow!* Pain is a brain perception, so the particular area in the brain that represents your finger pain actually increases in size; it processes the perception of pain differently. This is because your brain wants feedback on the finger to ensure that everything is okay. The more you worry about your finger (*Will it ever stop bleeding? Will it get infected?*), the more sensitive that area of the brain gets. It is similar to an important news story: big news, more journalists reporting on the issue. After injury, in this heightened state of awareness, people tend to be hypersensitive to pain. In fact, when you're on high alert, even looking at your finger can trigger a pain sensation. But the less you worry about your finger (*It's clotting already. The cut's not that bad.*), the smaller that area of the brain becomes. As the injury heals and your fear recedes, that area of the brain will return to its original size.

Pain can be frightening. The thought of losing the ability to do what you love to do, let alone the fear that this unpleasant sensation will never go away, can be overwhelming. Discovering the root of your pain isn't always as simple as completing a one-page questionnaire. But paying attention, using your emotions to problem-solve, and taking control of what you can are the first steps toward finding the imbalance in the body and feeling better.

I encourage you to develop a relationship with your body's sensations. I have been amazed over the years at the difference between two patients with identical structural pathology but differing beliefs about their injury. When a patient accepts their body's condition, learns what is safe to do, and the next steps they have to take, they tend to recover and return to excellent and usually pain-free function. Others cannot seem to help themselves, literally and figuratively speaking. Their pain experience becomes very emotional and does not allow them to connect with their body. They fail to take charge and guide their body into action. Because these patients believe that they are permanently injured, they remain in pain, unable to do certain activities.

The more familiar you become with the various sensations of pain, the better you will know how to interpret the body's message. Remember that pain is a warning, and if you listen, you can give your body what it needs to remain balanced. Pain is not necessarily a message to stop, but it is clearly a message to change, and that may involve changing both physically and emotionally.

This understanding of pain is not only useful for you; it's for your doctor, physiotherapist, massage therapist, and anyone else helping with your pain. We are all body detectives, and the more clues you give us, the easier it will be to solve the mystery of your pain.

Knowing how to describe pain, and what different pains mean, is a great start. But what other information do you need to take to your caregivers to help reach the proper diagnosis and create a treatment plan?

Getting a Checkup

Everybody has a different threshold for pain, and I have been amazed over the years at the differences. One patient with a completely normal physical examination feels completely debilitated, while another person who has lost range of motion and demonstrates complete joint destruction on an X-ray has almost no pain. It is fascinating to me and a testament to the complexity of our personal experience of pain.

If you are unsure whether your pain merits a trip to the doctor's office, you probably should go and get a checkup. Not every single little ache or muscle twitch is an emergency, but if you have pain that is interfering with your function, and particularly if you have any of the associated symptoms we will discuss below, then you should go see a doctor, particularly those with pain above a 4 on the NPRS. While the focus of this book is pain rooted in an active lifestyle and musculoskeletal wear and tear, pain can be a manifestation of a much more serious problem, even something potentially life-threatening like cancer. If that's the case, you want to know so you can treat it. If that's not the case, you want to know so you can rule it out and relax.

When I tell my patients that their pain isn't life-threatening and it's going to improve, they start to feel better right away. Knowledge brings hope, and hope helps relieve suffering. By recognizing that our injuries are treatable, we can stop worrying and start working.

How I Make a Diagnosis

Pain is just one of the symptoms we listen to as doctors. Understanding your own pain and communicating effectively about it with your treatment team are important in establishing the right diagnosis. I make a diagnosis from the history of the pain, the physical examination findings, and then any special tests such as blood work or radiographs. In addition to the qualities of pain that we've discussed, a doctor needs to know specific details about your pain.

- Where is the pain located? If you don't know the name of the body part, just point to it.
- Describe your pain. Some common descriptors are sharp, dull, crampy, achy, shooting, stabbing, throbbing, or burning. Any word that comes to mind is okay. It is your pain after all.
- How long have you had the pain? "Not long" or "A long time" can mean different things to different people, so give the best number you can. For example, one week or one year.
- How bad is the pain? Use the NPRS to describe your pain at its best and worst. (0 is no pain, while 10 is the worst pain imaginable.)
- Is the pain constant, or does it come and go?
- What makes it better? Or worse?

Often times, it is tricky to describe what you are feeling. You know that something is off or not right—you feel funny. There is no right or wrong; your pain is your pain. I have always said that patients know best. You and your body have the answers, so the better we can communicate, the easier it is for the doctor to solve the pain mystery. Help your doctor by becoming a body detective.

Initially, pain is telling us that something is out of balance in the body, and if you ignore the symptoms, it starts to break down. This is when associated symptoms develop. I always ask my patients about the following:

- **SWELLING** is to me the most sensitive sign of tissue damage. It's important to report how long the swelling has been there and note if it goes up and down or is always present.
- **RANGE OF MOTION** can indicate certain kinds of injuries, so any loss here is significant.
- **LOCKING** happens when something is caught in the joint, like a stone in your shoe. The loose tissue, often called "joint mice," is often a piece of bone or cartilage that can move around. One minute, the mouse is hiding in a corner; the next, it is at the joint surface blocking motion. If something

is mechanically stopping the joint from moving, we often have to remove it surgically. If your joint is "locked," you have to stop what you are doing and give the joint a little jiggle. There should be a sensation of release, and you can move again. Sometimes, a piece of tissue is not completely loose but is preventing movement because it's torn and jammed between the joint surface—for example, a piece of torn cartilage in the knee (meniscus). Locking is different from catching. Sometimes when you move, you may experience a sudden catch, jump, or clicking feeling. This happens if a tight piece of tissue moves over a bony prominence and does not actually stop the joint from moving. Always tell your doctor if locking or catching is happening. It can be painful, though sometimes it is not.

- **GIVING WAY** is when an arm or leg suddenly buckles. Make a note of what you are doing when this happens. Common examples of when someone's knee gives way are walking downstairs and changing direction when chasing a ball. Swelling often accompanies giving way, so I ask about that here too.

- **NOISY JOINTS** are common as we get older. Snaps, crackles, and pops in our joints can be noisy, but I do not usually worry about them unless they are associated with locking or an acute injury. Even though most noises are painless and benign, I mention them as many people find them unnerving. Whether they point to a serious injury or not, they're worth discussing.

More generally, red flags are symptoms that doctors always want to know about: if you are feeling generally unwell, have lost weight, have a fever, have a decrease in appetite, lost control of your bowel or bladder, or lost control of your limbs (paralysis). These symptoms can signal more serious medical conditions such as a disc herniation with pressure on nerve roots, cancer, or infection. Always report these symptoms to your doctor right away.

Special Investigations

Once your health care provider has listened to you (at least I hope they have) and performed an examination, they may want to get some special investigations such as blood work, X-rays, or an MRI to name a few. These tests will provide additional information to support a diagnosis. *But whatever you do, please do not rely too heavily on the result of an MRI!*

Our body does not have to be perfect to be pain free. Many times, an MRI shows us tears that have developed slowly over time, and the person had no idea that there was a problem. I am fascinated by the number of people with full thickness rotator cuff tears or with disc herniations who have functioned for years with no clue that their shoulder or back had any structural deficiencies. Numerous studies have been performed on asymptomatic people to determine the normal incidence of various pathologies. There is an age-related increase in degenerative changes. For example, disc degeneration increases from an incidence of 37 percent in one's 20s to 68 percent in one's 40s to 93 percent in one's 70s. The incidence of disc herniation, commonly known as a slipped disc, has a similar age-related incidence, with 40 percent of the population having a herniation in their 70s. These issues we see on MRIs are in people with zero back pain! Given how common degenerative changes are, we need to be sure that what is observed on the MRI is the cause of the current symptoms. If there is some wear and tear identified on an MRI, your physician should correlate the history of pain, other associated symptoms, and the physical examination findings to be clear that the pathology identified is indeed causing your pain. Clearly, we don't operate on half of the population, nor should we.

I've said this many times: We do not treat X-rays or MRIs. We treat people. I'm amazed at the number of times I have seen a patient with a terrible-looking X-ray but minimal symptoms; or the reverse, a normal radiograph and debilitating pain. The take-home message is to be sure the MRI abnormality is the root cause of your pain so that you get the correct treatment.

Make Pain Your Ally

We have a saying in tennis: "Make the wind your ally." While wind can be endlessly frustrating to a beginner player, it doesn't have to be. If you understand how the wind affects the ball, you can use it to your advantage.

The same is true of pain. If we can learn what our pain is trying to tell us, we can make pain our ally. Of course, this is not to suggest we shouldn't alleviate our pain—far from it. But to alleviate our pain, we must first understand what it's trying to say. *Have I just worked out too hard and have DOMS, or have I done something to my knee?* In the case of wear and tear injuries, pain is a signal for change, a sign that you need to adjust what you are doing, make two trips to carry your groceries instead of one. Pain provides amazing feedback, telling us that we are overloading some part of our musculoskeletal system, either metabolically (not enough oxygen or fuel) or mechanically (too much tension or compression). Learning to listen to the language of pain is the first step to alleviate your symptoms.

MOVEMENT MESSAGES

- Pain is the body's voice telling you something has to change.
- Learn the language of your pain. If you are unsure, see your doctor to determine if your pain is protecting you or telling you that there is pathology.
- Pain won't kill you, but lack of motion will. Develop a relationship with your pain. Listening to your body and changing how you move by using pain as feedback will give you control over your life.

CHAPTER 3

Using Movement as Medicine

We all know how good movement is for our heart, lungs, brain, and, of course, our muscles. We need to move to live. Moving when you have a solid foundation gives the cells in your body purpose, keeps them alive and strong. But moving poorly without a foundation can create problems. Every day, our bodies must contend with thousands of different challenges from high-pressure deadlines at work that leave us tense to workouts or physical tasks that leave our muscles exhausted. Even little movements, like carrying your purse or picking up your toddler, have an impact on your body. These day-to-day stresses create wear and tear on our musculoskeletal system. Without proper rest and care, this wear and tear accumulates, slowly morphing into imbalances and full-blown injuries. Dumping garbage into a truck for a day will leave you sore; doing it for three decades without a proper foundation can leave you incapacitated. We tend to think that the day we feel pain is the day the injury happened; in reality, the damage is usually due to a lifetime of injury that was not adequately repaired. If we understand how movement leads to our body's deterioration, we can then change how we move to allow healing and repair. That is the beauty of our body: We *can* heal if we create a good Foundation for Movement.

For athletes or people with physical jobs, these daily challenges are even more pronounced. Consider all the muscles involved in throwing a football. You generate power with your legs and the quick rotation of your upper body, then you use the smaller muscles in your shoulder, elbow, and hand to fine-tune the ball's direction and release. Every link in this chain of movement is stressed during every throw, and after doing it hundreds of thousands of times, tension builds, imbalances develop, muscles fatigue, and eventually they stop working properly. This leads to micro-injuries that if neglected over time will lead to tissue breakdown and a loss of your Foundation for Movement. If, however, you allow your body to recover and you maintain a good Foundation for Movement, you can keep moving forever.

Thankfully, our bodies aren't helpless. Given the proper time and care, the body can repair itself to a remarkable degree, and so long as the injury that occurs in a day is repaired at night, no significant deterioration in our structure occurs. The single most important factor in injury prevention and movement longevity is proper recovery from your daily activities. How we rest has a major impact on how we heal.

Understanding the Imbalances in Our Body

Imbalances change how a joint is aligned and get in the way of its normal course of motion. An imbalance occurs when the soft tissues are too tight or the muscles aren't working properly. Imbalances can develop as a result of repetitive motions, including many of the ordinary day-to-day movements you never think about, like weeding the garden or clicking your mouse. Unless you're ambidextrous, you're probably performing these movements with only the dominant side of your body. If you're left-handed, you use your left hand to eat, your left arm to open a door, and your left leg to kick a ball. Even when you're doing something as simple as walking up the stairs, more often than not you'll lead with your dominant leg. Because our musculoskeletal system remodels based on the way in which it's stressed and loaded, these repetitive motions quite literally change the shape and structure of our bones and soft tissues over time, making it almost impossible to avoid imbalances, especially for those of us who play sports or have physically demanding jobs. The difference created from the actions we perform with each side of our body is even more extreme.

Imbalances also develop when we move without engaging the proper muscles. This is a self-perpetuating cycle with poor joint alignment or posture leading to poor movement patterns that often get worse over time. A change in the alignment of a joint changes the length of the muscles around the joint, and if a muscle is not at its optimal length, it does not work properly, which leads to a poor movement pattern. For example, if you spend eight hours a day at your desk with your head jutted over your chest as you type, you're going to develop an imbalance in your upper trapezius (or traps). Why? Over time, the cervical spine hyperextends as your chin juts forward and the base of your skull almost sits on your shoulders. As this poor posture slowly evolves, the muscles at the front of your neck lengthen, while those at the back become shorter. When muscles are not at their optimal resting length, they do not work as well, so other muscles (in this case, the upper traps) have to take over and compensate. When your head is leaned forward at your desk, the only muscles holding it up are the traps. The average human head weighs ten pounds, and when your traps are forced to hold it up without the help of your deep neck stabilizers, core, and back, they become overworked, tightening and shortening in response. It's like the difference between eight people trying to lift up a car versus one. All that weight was never meant for just one to hold.

Over time, as imbalances evolve and deepen, the way you use your muscles will change. Stabilizer muscles (which provide support and control balance) will start to go to sleep, forcing prime mover muscles (the bigger muscles like your trapezius and levator scapulae) to take over. The body adapts because it desperately wants to keep moving, but these adaptations force muscles to perform duties they weren't meant to. And so, because our musculoskeletal system is interconnected, one imbalance leads to another, which leads to another, and so on.

Eventually, some imbalances become permanent, which is to say you will no longer be able to correct the imbalance by contracting your muscles. This can happen for a variety of reasons, which include a change in the shape of one of the vertebrae or bones as a result of a fracture, degenerative arthritis, or other developmental conditions. In these cases, it is important to try to improve your posture—even by a few degrees—and maintain the ability to isometrically activate the surrounding muscles, as this can make a difference to the segments above and below the area that is degenerative and how much pain you ultimately experience.

Detecting Imbalances

You can detect imbalances in your body by looking for asymmetries. Sometimes, these asymmetries are perfectly natural. For example, our dominant side tends to be roughly 10 percent stronger than our non-dominant side, so it's normal to see a slight discrepancy in muscle size. What you want to be on the lookout for are bigger discrepancies in muscle development and range of motion. For instance, if you're looking in the mirror as you brush your teeth, you might notice that one shoulder sits lower than the other. If so, probe further. Do you have limited range of motion in one of the shoulders? Does it feel different?

Later in the book, we'll look at how to perform a movement screen: a system for scanning yourself to pick up many of your imbalances in mobility or strength. For now, it's enough to keep in mind that finding these imbalances allows you to fix them before they become injuries.

That being said, if you are already in pain, don't rely on self-diagnosis alone. Our bodies may have hundreds of different imbalances, many of which are subtle and hard to detect, especially when you're investigating your own body. It's great if you can detect an imbalance, but if you want to be really thorough or are suffering pain, it's worth consulting a professional.

When the Body Can't Catch Up

With proper rest and nutrition, your body will heal itself. But if it isn't given enough time to fully heal, more activity can lead to more damage. Let's say that a runner who typically enjoys a five-kilometre run a few times each week decides one day to run a marathon instead of just five kilometres. This puts a lot of additional stress on her Achilles tendon, which attaches her calf muscle to her heel and contracts with every step. That night, the macrophage—a type of white blood cell that removes dead cells from the body and stimulates the action of other immune system cells—tosses away the broken collagen resulting from the additional load on the Achilles, and some new replacement collagen gets pumped in. But here's the problem: The job doesn't get finished. There was just too much to do. If only 60 percent of the ruptured collagen was repaired, that's not the end of the world; it will keep healing in the following days. But what if the runner runs another marathon the very next day, and another one the day after that? When the body can't repair the damaged tissue fast enough, and wear and tear builds, one day a minor misstep causes the Achilles tendon to finally tear.

This is an extreme example. Wear and tear can occur over years—even decades—and you likely won't even know it's happening. It's not until there's a critical threshold in tissue damage that inflammation becomes pathological and pain develops.

Pain and the Inflammatory Merry-Go-Round

Inflammation is the body's attempt to heal an internal wound, a normal response to tissue injury. Whenever our immune system detects damage, the cells of the immune system sweep in to repair the area. If, however, the repair process is incomplete before more damage occurs, inflammation develops. Inflammation is normal wound healing that has gone off the rails, so the key is to help the body do what it is meant to, which is finish the repair process.

A typical sequence in the repair process has a few steps. First, removing the damaged tissue. Second, laying down a new matrix for specialized cells to secrete protein. And third, remodelling, maturation, and strengthening of regenerated tissue. The initial repair tissues are fragile and need time to mature and become strong. If you continue to overload the tissues before they have matured during the regenerative process, your body will break down again, and signs of inflammation (such as swelling), loss of motion, and feelings of stiffness will occur. We are spinning our wheels, so to speak, because we have not found our rhythm for recovery. To prevent degeneration, we need to give our body time to heal.

When the body can't catch up and a repetitive cycle of injury and attempted repair occurs, chronic inflammation often develops. This is the inflammatory merry-go-round. Inflammation occurs when the normal cycle of repair or wound healing is continuously interrupted, so cell signals get mixed up and the healing process has to start all over again. The swelling associated with inflammation can be painful and can prevent normal function of the local tissues, leading to loss of motion, inhibition of muscle function, tissues adhering to one another, and excessive fibrosis. This perpetuates the wear and tear problem because it creates more imbalance and muscle compensation. The tissues become less pliable and stiff, making them tougher to rebalance. The changes in length of the muscles, tendons, and fascial connections alter the way the joints and tissues are loaded, and the body becomes more susceptible to localized wear and tear.

It is so important to control inflammation. You can use a combination of rest, anti-inflammatory treatments (such as ice), ultrasound, laser or acupuncture, and diet.

If you have visible swelling, you should go to the doctor, who can rule out other causes of inflammation, such as autoimmune disorders (rheumatoid arthritis or ankylosing spondylitis), infection (bacterial or fungal), and metabolic conditions (such as gout). Once other causes of inflammation are excluded, it is most likely that the chronic inflammation was caused by degenerative wear and tear, resulting in tissue breakdown and incomplete healing. Rest will often decrease the inflammation, but we must not forget why the inflammation developed in the first place: mechanical overload of the tissues as a result of imbalances and adaptive muscle-firing patterns. We have to address the inflammation and allow the body to repair itself, regaining normal tissue pliability, but if we don't also change how we are loading the body, the problem will just come back.

THE FOUR PHASES OF RECOVERY

1. **VASCULAR RESPONSE:** Damaged tissue leads to vasodilation. You may notice the area is red and warmer because the blood vessels have become larger in diameter and more permeable to allow healing cells and molecules to cross into the area more easily.
2. **INFLAMMATORY RESPONSE:** White blood cells, such as neutrophils and macrophages, enter the area of injury and remove the damaged tissue.
3. **TISSUE REPAIR:** Precursor cells differentiate into the specific tissue cell—for example, osteoblast (bone cell)—and begin to secrete a new tissue matrix to build a scaffold to repair the injured area.
4. **MATURATION AND REMODELLING:** The newly secreted matrix molecules mature and become stronger so that they are properly aligned and gain mechanical strength.

Injury Impact

It is important to understand the functional implications of an injury. We also need to understand whether there is a micro-injury that can heal without intervention, a partial injury at risk of progressing, or a complete tear of the tissues that cannot heal on its own. Can we function normally despite having this structural flaw? Just because it's broken doesn't mean we have to fix it. Is there something we can do to help the tissue to heal on its own? If not, can we stop further deterioration and learn to compensate for the loss of that structure?

We can often function despite a little—or even a lot of—wear and tear on our musculoskeletal system. Our bodies were made with backup plans, so when we don't listen to our pain and change how we move, we often compensate, and our wear and tear injuries continue to progress. As long as those compensations don't create new long-term problems, we can function well like this, and we may remain pain free regardless of the status of the tissue. Isn't that the goal—pain-free function? The important point here is to not get hung up on the fact that you have a structural injury. The damage is telling you that you need to change how you are loading that part of your body. The core message is to restore a Foundation for Movement by changing how you move; that will allow for healing or at least stop the degenerative process. The focus is on re-establishing pain-free function.

How Do You Move? Are You a Tortoise or a Hare?

The more intense the physical activity, the greater the stress on your musculoskeletal system, the more you'll exacerbate whatever musculoskeletal problem may already exist, and the more quickly an injury will likely progress. The physical demands of a construction worker, for instance, are very different from those of an accountant, and this can have a significant impact when dealing with wear and tear injuries.

Think of your body as a rope: strong in some places and fraying in others. Now think of physical activities as a series of weights: light for activities that cause little mechanical stress, and heavy for the ones that cause a lot. If you were to take a weight no heavier than a feather, you could place it anywhere on the rope, even the part where it's most heavily frayed, without a problem. But what happens when you use a 50-pound weight? If you place it on the sturdiest part of the rope, there would be no problem, but if you place it where the rope is fraying, it will fall apart faster, maybe even snap instantly. The way we load our musculoskeletal system affects not only how injuries develop but how they worsen.

The acuteness of the injury also determines whether there is a chance to adapt. A tendon that tears slowly over 50 years doesn't have the same impact as a tendon that tears with one movement. In fact, people with gradual tears often don't even notice them. This is because the body has compensated for the initial wear and tear injury, and other tissues share the load and protect the injured area whether the original injury heals or not. However, over time, we get to the point where our body can no longer compensate, and that's when the pain begins. This is why it can be such a challenge to undo

40 years of imbalances. It takes time, patience, and understanding of how to remodel movement and recover. But pain-free movement can be accomplished if we understand how the original problem began and then reverse it so that the tissues can heal.

The Rhythm of Recovery

The key to staying healthy is to detect your imbalances while they can still be corrected. Every day will lead to a small imbalance somewhere in your body, but if every day you do something to correct this imbalance, then serious issues are not as likely to develop.

If you consider the human body on a microscopic level, you will find it is in a constant cycle of injury and repair. If a molecule is damaged, that molecule can be replaced. If there are little tears in the proteins, they can be filled. Another way to think of the fascia is like a piece of fabric, or clothing, that encases our bones and tissues. The tiny threads that make up clothing are like the molecules of protein that make up our connective tissues. One of the most common connective tissue molecules is collagen. Now imagine your favourite pair of jeans that you wear every day for years. At first you may notice that a few threads of the fabric have thinned out, and eventually there is a small tear or hole. This is exactly what happens in our body. The major difference is that we have an internal seamstress. Our fascia is under constant surveillance by our immune system. Micro-injuries are detected and repaired on a daily basis. In fact, our entire collagen network is replaced every two years, bit by bit. Unlike a pair of jeans, our bodies don't just wear out. We are our own tailors, and wherever there's a blood supply, there's an opportunity for repair. The rhythm of recovery is balanced when any daily breakdown quickly gets repaired and we maintain the status quo. If you have overstressed your system and your body cannot repair all of the daily wear and tear, your rhythm of recovery goes into a deficit. Most of us can get away with some degree of deficit for days, weeks, and sometimes even years, but persistent and consistent breakdown will eventually lead to issues with our tissues. We can, however, regenerate if we build more tissue than we break down.

Our Connective Tissues Change to Suit Our Needs

Right after my second child was born, I thought I should do some sit-ups to get my core strong again. As I proceeded to perform a crunch, I was horrified and bewildered to see a giant hernia appear on my abdomen! I was so shocked and cried out, "What the heck was that!" I realized that the fascia between my abdominal muscles (rectus abdominis) had stretched during pregnancy. The tissue had to lengthen to accommodate the presence of a baby (and a large one at that, almost ten pounds), but now that there was no baby in my abdomen, there was all of this "extra" tissue. The fascia between our rectus muscles is normally about one or two fingertips in width; after my pregnancy, I could actually place my fist between the rectus muscles! This is a common condition affecting women after pregnancy and is known as a diastasis recti.

It was not painful, although I suffered from some back and pelvic pain due to my weak core. I was so busy with two kids under the age of two and returning to my surgical practice (I got six weeks of maternity leave) that I did not have time to think about the hernia. Consistent with my general attitude toward life, I put my head down and moved. I did my core exercises and carried on with life. I honestly cannot remember exactly how much time passed, but one day I realized the hernia was gone! Now I can only fit one fingertip between my abdominals. This was a huge revelation with regards to the remodelling capacity of our body. Over the course of about a year, the tissue between my rectus muscles had literally shortened by four centimetres.

My experience highlights one of the most important principles for healing and recovering from wear and tear injuries: Our tissues will remodel to meet the needs of the body, making more tissue if space or strength is required and removing tissue that is unnecessary or unused. Stressing the tissues in the right way can repair the issues. This is how movement becomes medicine!

Muscle Activation Is Key

Scientific studies have clearly shown that our connective tissues all remodel based upon the stress that is applied. We can strengthen tissues that need strengthening if we move properly. Similar to the way our bodies respond by creating extra tissue when under stress, they also respond to the way we move our bodies during repair.

Let's say you tore a muscle in your right thigh. If you keep that leg absolutely still for 15 days, you'll end up with a mess of scar tissue where the tear used to be. Why? Because when that muscle isn't being stressed, the body doesn't know how to rebuild it. Mechanical stressors are like the directions in an instruction manual. Without them, the body is lost. If you lightly stress that torn muscle in your right thigh, you'll send the body the information it needs to properly rebuild.

Muscle activation is key. At first, it should be only isometric movement, which means contracting the muscles without moving the joint. Think of holding something in place. The contraction sends a signal to the cells directing the healing response but does not change the length of the muscle, meaning there is no disruption of the healing tissue. The isometric muscle contraction also pumps any unwanted fluid and waste products out of the injury area, which has a positive effect on decreasing fibrosis (scarring or thickening of the tissue), decreasing pain, and maintaining mobility.

This process requires real balance and delicacy. With no mechanical stress, a tear will fill with disorganized scar tissue. With too much mechanical stress, the tear won't heal—or, worse, will tear again. The trick is to tread lightly. Remember: enough but not too much. Let's examine this in more detail by understanding what our Foundation for Movement is and how to get one.

MOVEMENT MESSAGES

- Injuries ranging from micro to macro are a normal part of life.
- The earlier an imbalance is identified, the easier it is to correct. Even chronic imbalances can be fixed.
- Our body is alive, and injuries can heal. How we heal depends on how we move.
- Become familiar with your rhythm of recovery. Listen to it so you can give it what it needs.
- Don't stop moving; just change how you move!

PART II

Healing with Movement

CHAPTER 4

Building a Foundation for Movement

There is a movement hierarchy in life. To move with speed, for instance, we require strength. But before we attempt to enhance our movements for increased performance, there is a necessary foundation that must be in place. To have strength, for example, we need to have good mobility and stability of our joints. To help explain this concept, I developed the Foundation for Movement and the Performance Pyramid. They evolved out of my work with professional athletes but apply to anyone and everyone with wear and tear pain.

Before we focus on enhancing our movements for increased performance (see Chapter 10), there is a necessary base, or foundation, that must be in place. This foundation consists of tissue quality, activation of the correct muscles throughout each movement, alignment of our joints, and having a full active range of motion (ROM). Once you have your foundation, you can begin to progress up the Performance Pyramid, progressively increasing stress on the body to enhance your functional mobility. We'll focus more on the pyramid in Chapter 10, but for now it's helpful to know that the rate at which you progress up the pyramid—adding endurance, strength, power, and speed—and remain pain free depends on your ability to maintain your foundation.

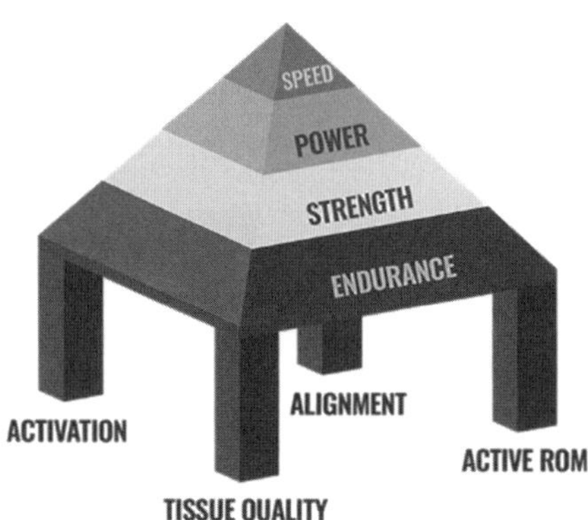

In this chapter, we will focus on the four key pillars of your Foundation for Movement. Only when all four pillars are in place is the pyramid stable. And it is only when the pyramid is stable—when we have a solid Foundation for Movement—that we are able to enhance our everyday movements in ways that will not lead to injury. At the top of the pyramid is the activity you wish to perform, whether that is a recreational activity, your job, housework—anything.

Have you ever been so strapped for time that you try to clean the house in a nanosecond? You're between school pickup, grocery shopping, and making dinner, vacuuming at the speed of light, when you bend down to get under the couch and whammy—your back goes into spasm? The result may have been very different if you had vacuumed leisurely on a Sunday morning and slowly bent down to retrieve that dust bunny. Everyone must have a Foundation for Movement in order to stay healthy and active.

The reality is most people don't have a Foundation for Movement. Even the professional athletes that I examine—all of them could work on their foundation! Living life and being active leads to an almost daily loss of some part of our foundation. Some days we lose more than others. Learning about our rhythm of recovery—the amount of time it takes for our bodies to repair themselves—and how we can restore our Foundation for Movement with some simple exercises is key. Just like brushing our teeth every day, we need to maintain our bones and joints to keep them healthy.

Over the years, I have learned there are two reasons people experience wear and tear pain. The first is that someone doesn't have a Foundation for Movement. Trying to do an activity that requires strength or speed without the foundation will overload the musculoskeletal system, subjecting it to wear and tear. If you can't do a simple squat because you have a stiff ankle, putting weight on your back is not going to help! Picture a table with only three legs—in this case, proper range of motion is the missing leg: It cannot be stable, and that leads to increased stress on the tissues. The goal of this book is to teach you how to obtain and maintain your foundation for pain-free movement.

As we know, when the musculoskeletal system is overloaded, it breaks down and eventually inflammation and pain develop. This is a good news–bad news situation. The good news is that it often takes years for the body to break down. The bad news is that as the years go by, the compensations become more ingrained, and it takes time to progress through the restoration and remodelling of your body. Most people (including me) want instant results.

The second reason for wear and tear happens on the pyramid: The individual has a good Foundation for Movement but jumps too high up the pyramid, trying to perform in a manner that their body is not prepared for. Imagine trying to throw a 100 mile-per-hour fastball when you don't have enough strength. You can't cheat the system. If you skip up the pyramid too quickly, trying to run before you can crawl, pain will develop.

It's impossible to live life without developing wear and tear on our musculoskeletal system. And while rest is crucial for resolving micro-injuries and remodelling our bones and soft tissue, rest alone isn't always enough. If you don't address the reasons why the tissues were overly stressed—such as postural imbalances or muscles that are tight or weak—pain will recur shortly after resuming your activity. With this in mind, I have developed a two-pronged approach to wear and tear injuries. Phase 1 teaches you how to establish a Foundation for Movement, and Phase 2 provides you with the principles for progression through the Performance Pyramid so you can safely return to or excel in your activity. It may take time, but slow and steady wins the race. The rest of this chapter is devoted to Phase 1; we delve into Phase 2 in Chapters 5 to 9.

Phase 1: The Four Pillars of the Foundation for Movement

PILLAR 1: TISSUE QUALITY

When a cycle of breakdown and interrupted repair progresses to chronic inflammation, the repeated attempts to regenerate tissue can cause poor tissue elasticity. The tissues can "stick" together. Muscles, tendons, and fascia do not move with their usual suppleness and lose their normal function. That loss affects the alignment and mobility of the neighbouring joints and interferes with the ability of the adjacent muscles to work properly. With tight or restricted tissues come weak muscles. Since tissue quality has such a profound impact on our musculoskeletal function, one of the first goals is to restore a healthy connective tissue environment.

What do we mean by poor tissue quality? There is a spectrum that goes from dehydrated, inflamed, fibrotic, tight, stiff, and non-pliable tissues to a partial tear and finally to full damage of the musculoskeletal structure. Tissues that are overused and abused cannot recover and so become stiff, non-pliable structures that break down. If there is complete structural breakdown, like a tear in a muscle or tendon or a fractured bone, we need to know if that tissue has the capacity to heal on its own or if a cast or surgery is required. You should see your doctor for direction.

You don't have to wait for your tissues to break down before you do something about their quality. Often, we are not aware that there is a problem. This is where identifying compensations early can allow you to address the root cause of your issue before pain even develops. We can take steps every day to keep our body as healthy as possible. All the little things you heard growing up really work: eat right, drink plenty of water, get enough exercise and a good sleep. These behaviours help to supply all of the necessary building blocks for normal repair and remodelling. Hydration, in particular, is a key component to tissue quality that is commonly neglected.

If you have an injury, then we need to break the wear and tear cycle by promoting an environment for regeneration and recovery. We do this by taking the mechanical load off the abnormal tissue: not completely, but enough to stop the tissue breakdown. We must work to decrease swelling and improve tissue hydration, so the tissue has time to heal and restore its normal quality.

There are several recovery scenarios that depend on the quality of your tissues. If you have tightness, and the tissues are otherwise intact with no significant inflammation, performing active self-myofascial release (ASMR), like foam rolling, combined with isometric muscle activation will quickly correct your problem and allow you to restore full mobility. Generally, people who fall into this category respond very well to a simple change in movement patterns. Once the correct muscles are engaged, the stiff and sore ones can relax. Once they relax, joint alignment and mobility is restored, and activities can be resumed.

For those with a partial tear and inflammation, we need to break the cycle of inflammation and activate all the proper muscles using a combination of rest, modalities (ice, heat, ultrasound, or laser, for example), possibly medication, and a modified form of ASMR (no foam rolling directly on the injured area). Performing ASMR on an acutely torn muscle or tendon will continuously disrupt the body's attempt to fix it. I look at the area or zone of injury as the centre of a bull's eye. You can release tissues far away from the bull's eye to take pressure off the area while it is trying to heal. As the injury begins to resolve and the healing tissue matures, the ASMR can move closer to the centre ring until it's safely right on target.

Releasing tension on damaged tissue through ASMR allows the tissues to repair and regenerate and, over time, return to normal. Usually, if there is a tear and some inflammation, it will take six weeks to see a fundamental change in the tissue pliability. If it happens sooner, fantastic, but you need to be mentally prepared for it to take some time for your body to repair the damaged area.

In situations where there is complete disruption of the tendon, muscle, or bone, a surgical consultation may be required to determine if the structure can heal with simple rest or immobilization. As surgeons, we recognize specific patterns of injury. There are several variables that come into play when making a decision to operate. Creating as much good tissue as possible will help you recover faster, regain better function, and prevent the surgical repair from suffering the same fate as the original damaged tissue.

PILLAR 2: ACTIVATION

Think of an inactive muscle as someone who's fallen asleep or a machine that's powered off. It's not dead or broken; it just needs to be woken up or turned on. Like people, our muscles can be in different stages of sleep. Sometimes all it takes is a few light taps to wake a muscle up. But for a muscle that's been inactive for weeks, months, or years, it takes more effort. It's important to reactivate these muscles because waking them up breaks our compensatory movement patterns.

Let's look at the gluteal muscles (read: butt) as an example. If you spend all day sitting, they shut off. You might be thinking, *So what? Let my glutes take some time off. They've earned it!* Well, when you finally do stand up and start walking around, your butt might've been inactive for so long that it fails to wake up. To compensate, your hamstrings are forced to pull double duty, doing their job and that of the glutes. As you might've guessed, this isn't great for the hamstrings, which can grow so overworked they become taut. That limits your range of motion and changes the alignment of your pelvis.

Inactive muscles are also common after acute injuries. For instance, if you have an acute injury that causes your knee to swell, your quadriceps will atrophy in response. I have observed significant muscle loss in less than 24 hours. This is why it's so important to keep the local muscles awake after injury or surgery. The sooner you reactivate them, the less they'll atrophy. Just remember: enough but not too much.

In principle, reactivating your muscles is as simple as waking them up and getting them firing again. However, this can be more challenging than it sounds, especially if the muscle hasn't been firing properly for a long time. Let's go back to the butt. The problem isn't so much turning it on; it's keeping it on. It's like a bad case of narcolepsy: The muscle wakes up only to fall right back to sleep.

The simplest way to activate your glutes is to consciously contract and relax the muscle over and over again. You can do this as you're lying face down on a yoga mat or when you're standing in line at the bank. If you try to contract the muscle and can't do it, you're going to need to manually stimulate the area to get it firing again. Yes, this does mean repeatedly tapping your butt. And no, I don't recommend doing that in line at the bank. Take a break from sitting every hour to fire up your glutes. Gluteal amnesia is such a common problem because most of us spend a lot of time on our butts. Keeping the glutes active with a little reminder every hour can go a long way in preventing future compensations.

After you manually stimulate the area, try contracting and relaxing again. If it works, great. If not, go back to tapping. Learn to slowly ramp up the intensity of the contraction, with 0 being no contraction and 10 being maximum contraction. This is a great way to develop kinesthetic awareness—the ability to sense your body's position and movement—and the activation of your muscles. With this sense of control, when you have an injury, you can start with a low-intensity contraction to stimulate the tissues without pulling apart the repair.

The more conscious you are that a muscle is on or off, the better. At first, the muscle must be reminded to wake up often, but over time, once some endurance in the motor pattern is created, the activation becomes more automatic. Visualizing the anatomy of the muscle and understanding the motion you are trying to create with the muscle contraction can help reawaken your sleeping giants.

A key to maintaining proper balance around the joints and good tissue quality is to use proper movement patterns. Often when we try to perform an exercise or a specific movement, our brain defaults to the most recently used movement pattern; it can be a challenge to re-establish the proper muscle activation routine. For this reason, we use a movement technique known as dissociation, which resets the neuromuscular system by having you perform the opposite movement pattern to your habitual ones.

Try this: Push your ankle downward, like you're stepping on the gas pedal in a car. You probably automatically also pointed your toes instead of extending them toward your nose, yes? This is the normal movement pattern. If you have an injury in the lower extremity, in your knee, for example, we need to make sure the joints above and below it—the hip and the foot and ankle, in this case—are moving well and using the correct muscles. In order to do this, we need to uncouple or dissociate the usual movement patterns to awaken and activate the sleeping muscles. Try it. Dissociate the movement of your toes and ankle by pushing your ankle downward and this time extend your toes toward your nose while you do it. This will feel strange at first, but the more you do it, the more you become aware of how the muscles in your foot and ankle are working. If we don't break the movement down like this, it is too easy to use the same old habitual patterns, which perpetuates poor tissue quality and muscular inactivation and leads to recurrent problems.

Here is a very common issue I see in my clinical practice: You are prescribed a set of exercises by your therapist to strengthen a specific range of motion for a joint. You go home and do your exercises and either don't get better or feel more pain. This is because you have unconsciously continued to use the compensatory muscles. It's not your fault. This is your movement habit, the way your body and brain have been programmed to compensate. Unless we break down these movement compensations and become aware of what it feels like to contract a muscle we're not used to using, it is very difficult to re-establish proper movement patterns.

It's difficult at first, but it's important to become aware of how your body moves and which muscles are contributing to the motion. The dissociation exercises I teach later in the book will help you build this body awareness and reset your movement patterns, setting the stage for full mobility.

PILLAR 3: ALIGNMENT

After we gently release the tight non-pliable tissues from the area surrounding an injury, we can begin to restore proper joint alignment.

There are two distinct types of alignment: static alignment, which is akin to a neutral resting position of joints, and dynamic alignment, which is the ability to maintain optimal joint position when the joint is moving.

We can assess static alignment by looking at you from various angles. Spine, head, and neck posture is the most common representation of static alignment, but the positions of your knees, shoulder blades, and even what direction your palms face when your arms are down by your sides reveal the static alignment of your joints.

Dynamic alignment is more difficult to assess and requires a trained eye to detect alignment-related aberrations during movement. We often use the term *centration* when describing dynamic alignment, especially when referring to movements of the shoulders and hips, because we want the head of the limb (humerus and femur, respectively) to remain centred within its socket. Poor centration can lead to excess wear and tear on tendons and the joint surface, as well as impingement (compression of the tendon), eventually resulting in tissue damage and pain.

If a joint is centrated, it is perfectly aligned, so motion at the joint does not cause excessive stress on the surface or accessory structures (cartilage, meniscus, discs, and tendons). If, however, the joint is slightly misaligned, there will be asymmetrical loading of the joint cartilage, capsule, and ligaments, which over time makes them vulnerable to wear and tear. Even more important, when a joint is not balanced or centrated, the surrounding muscles will not be at their optimal length—they'll be either too long or too short. A muscle that doesn't maintain its normal resting length has trouble activating or turning on. And if a muscle doesn't turn on and work the way it's supposed to, an adjacent muscle will take over, and we have the start of compensation and movement dysfunction. Plus, the muscle that has stopped working no longer exerts pressure on its tendon, joint capsule, and fascia, and that causes the tissues to become stiff and weak. Proper alignment supports proper muscle activation. Both are critical to maintaining our Foundation for Movement.

The goal of maintaining good alignment is to re-establish shapes of resilience along the kinetic chain, keeping the tissues balanced and healthy. We know that movement at one joint affects movement at another. So, if there is a problem with joint alignment, mobility, or stability, there will be compensatory movement above or below that joint. A common example of poor alignment occurs at the foot and ankle. When the foot and ankle collapse inward, it causes the knee to be misaligned, and it will also start to collapse inward. Loss of alignment is associated with increased incidence of Achilles tendon (ankle tendon) and anterior cruciate ligament tears (the most common knee ligament injury). Fixing problems with alignment requires first waking up sleepy muscles, making them strong, and then integrating these muscles into various movement patterns. There are cues within many of the exercises in Chapters 5 to 9 that will help you restore optimal alignment for healthy, pain-free joints.

THE POWER OF ACTIVE STRETCHING

Static stretches are a form of passive stretching: when you stretch a muscle without active muscular contraction to hold you in the range of motion you're working. Take the hamstrings, for example. If you lie on your back with your legs extended and then grab the back of one thigh, pulling that straight leg toward your head, you will passively lengthen the hamstring. This can improve flexibility in your hamstring, but the lengthening is temporary, lasting only a few minutes or a few hours. This phenomenon occurs because our nervous system gets *nervous* when we have more range of motion but do not have the muscular control over the new length; it's an unstable situation. So, unless we can actively move the body through a range of motion, we lose it! Also, when we passively stretch, we move through the path of least resistance, often stretching already pliable tissues that don't need it, leaving the less pliable sections restricted.

Active stretching works differently: It stretches a muscle by using the opposing muscle group to actively pull it to its end range of motion. Try an active hamstring stretch by lying on your back: Lift your leg toward the ceiling, and push your knee straight using your quadriceps muscle. Active stretching does two things. First, in this example by activating the quadriceps muscle, we send a neurological signal to the hamstring to *relax*. Second, we send signals to the fibroblast cells—cells that create and maintain connective tissue—within the hamstring tendon, capsule, fascia, and muscle to *lengthen* and create permanent changes in the muscle quality. These signals are not sent when the hamstrings are stretched passively. The active movement of the body starts the lasting remodelling process.

PILLAR 4: ACTIVE RANGE OF MOTION

When it comes to improving your range of motion (ROM), most people think of flexibility and static stretching as the ideal means to improve it. It makes sense. Someone with great hip flexibility can sit in the middle splits, which is a common static stretch.

But if you're running around on the tennis court and you're forced to spread your legs similar to the middle splits (think Novak Djokovic) to return an opponent's shot out wide, the ability to do the split stretch doesn't necessarily translate to the court because it's missing the strength, speed, and power to get into and out of that position when you need to.

Flexibility allows a joint to be put into a certain range of motion, whereas mobility means a joint can enter, stabilize, and exit a range of motion. Put another way, flexibility is passive while mobility is active. That's why our fourth pillar is active range of motion (ROM), with the emphasis on *active*.

There are two pieces to this pillar. First is active muscular control of our full range of motion. When we perform static stretching, we're increasing range of motion passively without building any strength or stability. The increased range of motion thus has no active muscular support. That support won't magically appear out of nowhere; it needs to be trained. Increased range without strength is essentially instability, and instability is a common reason why joint structures like ligaments get damaged. This is why I avoid the classic passive static stretches that to this day are still seen as the go-to for improving range of motion. Instead, the exercises in this book prioritize active muscular control. You'll learn to perform them smoothly and slowly through a full range, without using any momentum.

Second, we need to ensure we have sufficient range of motion for the movements we perform in life, sport, and any recreational activities. If you're performing tasks where you have to reach up overhead—maybe a job that has you stocking shelves, or a strong serve if you play tennis—and you don't have the shoulder range of motion needed, you will compensate to get the job done.

In this case, the most common compensation for a lack of overhead shoulder range of motion is the lumbar spine. If this individual suffers from low back pain and their rehab doesn't address their insufficient shoulder range of motion, they'll never get lasting results. This is the kinetic chain in action. It illustrates how when we lose mobility in one area, other joints above and/or below compensate, increasing wear and tear. Building active range of motion through the full movements we perform is critical to preventing future wear and tear injuries.

End-Range Expansion

End-range expansion (ERE) techniques take advantage of several normal biological principles. You may have heard of proprioceptive neuromuscular facilitation stretching, which is a mouthful! This is the same thing with a simpler name. These techniques employ the one-on/one-off principle. If we want to lengthen a muscle on one side of the body, we can take advantage of the fact that contraction of the muscle on one side of the body will lead to reciprocal inhibition of the muscle and relaxation of the opposite. For example, if we want the biceps to lengthen, we can contract the triceps to move the elbow through a range of motion, and a neurological reflex will cause the biceps to relax, making it easier to lengthen the biceps. If we want to induce tissue remodelling, say lengthen a short biceps, actively pulling the tissue using your triceps muscle will cause the cells in the biceps to remodel along the lines of stress.

The major advantage of the ERE technique, however, is the development of strength at the end range of motion. Because we use our muscles actively to achieve the range, our brain learns that we are safe to use this range of motion. In other words, we "own" this new range of motion.

This is very different from what happens when you perform a static stretch or a therapist stretches your arm, which gives you temporary flexibility gains. Because you didn't use your muscles to move through the range, they will not be able to control the body in that new zone of mobility. No control means no stability—and no real improvement over time.

Getting Started: Re-establish Your Foundation for Movement

Understanding the four pillars of movement is a start toward creating a solid foundation of movement. But it's one thing to read about it and another to actually change the way you move. The real work lies ahead, and it requires you to take action!

There are a number of factors that will influence how quickly you recover from pain or injury. One important factor is how chronic your problem is. If the imbalance and compensation is relatively new and there is no tissue damage, the problem can be resolved within days, or even minutes. If, on the other hand, the imbalance and compensation have been present and slowly evolving over many years, it will take time for the connective tissue around the joint to become pliable and for you to establish new movement patterns and end-range motion. It may take weeks or months, and in the most difficult circumstances, it can take years to restore our four pillars. But the beauty of your body and mind is that with every little step you take to create a solid foundation, you will start to feel better. The work you put in today will give you a better tomorrow!

Even though it may take a long time to permanently remodel and restore your tissues, you will feel immediate benefits from doing the exercises in Chapters 5 to 9. For example, if you have a tight Achilles tendon, perhaps with some partial tearing, your pain will decrease from a 7 or 8 out of 10 to a 2 or 3 as soon as you perform ASMR of the tendon, followed by activation of the small intrinsic foot muscles and the hip muscles. You'll feel better because you are activating more of the muscle by doing these exercises. When you start to awaken your foot intrinsics, you may be recruiting only 50 percent of the muscle, but that is 50 percent more than when you began. After that, you will learn to recruit 80 to 90 percent, and this will make you stronger immediately.

Keep in mind that it takes four to six weeks for the muscle to truly become stronger from muscle hypertrophy (increased muscle mass). Simultaneously, while you are building stronger muscles, the Achilles tendon is repairing, so three of your pillars are moving in the right direction: tissue quality, muscle activation, and active range of motion. The more tissue that's damaged, the longer it takes for the body to repair, so a 30 percent partial tear will recover faster than a 70 percent partial tear. No matter how much damage there is, each step of the way is taking you closer to a solid Foundation for Movement, so please do not get discouraged. If you keep doing the right things, every six weeks will bring a big jump in how you feel. You may plateau for another six weeks, and then—*boom*—another noticeable improvement of your mobility and strength.

Most interesting to me is that the majority of patients report feeling better immediately after they activate the correct muscles. This is the power of motion. And while the old feelings of stiffness and pain may recur after lack of activity, those feelings diminish if you stick to the program. So, keep going. As you establish a foundation and strengthen it, your pain-free time will increase, and it will take more vigorous activity for symptoms to recur.

Don't forget: Our entire collagen network is replaced every two years, and each day is another opportunity to reprogram and remodel. Your body is constantly remaking itself, so why not direct how, so it does it better? This work requires commitment. But if you put in the work, you'll get the results.

The sequence of the four pillars is the key to treating and preventing wear and tear injuries for the long term. Once we have healthy pliable tissues, activate the correct muscles to move, align our body, and restore proper muscle activation through our full range of motion, we have established a Foundation for Movement. All four pillars are intact, and we have a solid tabletop! Understanding our individual rhythm of recovery, how quickly our tissues lose balance or our muscles fall asleep, is important. We need to develop daily habits to maintain our pillars, so the accumulation of everyday stress doesn't topple our foundation.

Depending on how you move, you will be more or less prone to developing movement imbalances and compensations. Catching these early and restoring your foundation are key to living a healthy life. We need motion in order to keep our tissues strong, healthy, and alive, but the very act of moving leads to the loss of our foundation. Spending

15 minutes every day on our foundation will go a long way in keeping us moving and pain free for life. Don't wait until you break down; do a little something every day to build yourself up! Training our fundamental movement patterns gets the kinetic chain working in sync, which allows us to work our way up the Performance Pyramid.

How to Use the Chapters That Follow

In Chapters 5 to 9, you will discover whether you have a Foundation for Movement in five key zones of the body: head, neck, and upper back; shoulders and arms; lower back and hips; knees; and ankles and feet. In my clinical observations over the past 30 years, these are the zones that tend to give people the most trouble. You will also learn some of the specific wear and tear consequences of not having a strong Foundation for Movement and how you can improve it in a targeted way.

Don't worry if you discover something is lacking. Actually, be thrilled if you identify things you can work on! It means you can get on the path to making improvements. Part of the reason I understand these imbalances so well is I have experienced all of them. Literally from the tip of the toes, starting with an ankle sprain as a teenager, to core issues after pregnancy and then shoulder problems during my tennis training. I have suffered from all of the classic wear and tear issues as a result of my imbalances, and wish I had known as a teenager what I know now. I believe I could have saved myself a lot of pain and time off from my activities. In each of the following chapters, I will share my personal experiences, where I had lost my foundation, what I felt, and how I recovered. I will also share some of my patients' experiences. You may not experience the same symptoms or problems that are presented in the examples that follow, but one thing is for sure: No matter what your underlying pain is, a Foundation for Movement needs to be re-established. Assessing each part of your body will give you a good sense of where to start.

If you find you have multiple zones that need to be corrected, I suggest starting by focusing on the area where you have pain. If you don't have pain, start with the area that is most imbalanced based on the assessments. From there, you can start to restore your Foundation for Movement with the simple exercise routine I provide at the end of each chapter. Remember, though, that we are connected from the tip of the toes to the tip of the nose. An imbalance in one part of the body means that compensations have had to occur elsewhere, so once you fix one area, you may need to move on to the next. If you are experiencing shoulder pain, for example, I recommend that you do the exercise routines written for the neck and for the back and hips as well. It's important not to neglect adjacent parts of the body because of the high probability that your foundation is starting to crumble along the kinetic chain—particularly if you have had a long-standing injury. For a well-rounded approach, you can cycle through each of the five zone-specific routines on a monthly basis and revisit the assessments periodically to monitor improvements and changes to your foundation.

MOVEMENT MESSAGES

- Our Foundation for Movement is defined by four interrelated pillars: tissue quality, activation, alignment, and active range of motion.
- Before you enhance your movements, the four pillars of your foundation must be in place.
- Once you have a strong foundation, you can start to increase stress on the body by adding endurance, strength, power, and speed.
- Imbalances can take anywhere from minutes to years to resolve. It depends on how chronic your problem is.
- Give to your body every day by spending a few minutes doing exercises that will restore your foundation.

CHAPTER 5

Head, Neck, and Upper Back

When we sit at our desk all day, drive for long distances, or, in my case, stand in the operating room for hours looking down into the surgical field, we can fall into the forward head posture trap. I did. I began to get upper back and neck pain, and my shoulder hurt while playing tennis.

What happened to me and my neck? Standing in the operating room for long periods of time, focused with my head looking down, created the conditions for wear and tear. As I got older and my eyesight grew worse, I had to lean forward even more. (Don't worry, I could still see clearly to operate.) That led to the development of even worse posture.

Our heads weigh about 10 to 12 pounds, and when we look down, the effect of gravity naturally pulls our chins closer to our chests. The problem is that for every inch that your head sits in front of your shoulder, the relative weight of the head increases by 10 pounds. When I assessed my own forward head posture, I found that it was sitting about three inches in front of my shoulders. Three inches equals a 42-pound head!

Allowing my head to sit forward meant I lost the alignment of my cervical and thoracic spine (where the neck and upper back meet), so one pillar of my foundation was gone. The cervical spine is connected to the thoracic spine; therefore, poor alignment of one affects the other. The thoracic spine connects to the ribs and the shoulder blades, so there is a domino effect with the forward head posture. The altered alignment affects the length of the muscles supporting the neck and shoulders. Some muscles cannot work properly, and so compensations develop. My upper traps and levator scapulae began to work overtime, and the deep stabilizing muscles of my neck, upper back, and shoulders (multifidus, lower traps, and serratus anterior) were not working well at all. No big deal if this happens for a day or two, but after weeks and months, even years in the OR, I developed tight traps and levator scapulae muscles because they were always having to work to hold up a head that felt much heavier than it actually is. Fewer muscles working to hold up a relatively heavier head means neck pain and sometimes even a headache. Eventually my neck got stiff, and I had trouble looking over my shoulder to check my blind spot while driving, and I was developing an impressive hunchback. That was a clue that I better get on top of my foundation of movement before I developed overloaded discs, nerve root compression, or arthritis.

DO YOU HAVE FORWARD HEAD POSTURE?

1. Stand up straight with your back against the wall with your heels, buttocks, and shoulders touching the wall. There should be a small space between the wall and your lower back. Tuck your chin and see if you can touch the back of your head to the wall. Keep your eyes looking straight ahead. If you have to tilt your chin up or you cannot touch the back of your head to the wall, you likely have forward head posture.

2. The other way to measure this is to take a picture of yourself from the side while standing naturally. Make sure that your shoulder, hip, and knees are aligned. Once you have the picture, draw a line from the middle of your ear straight down. This line should meet the centre of your shoulder. If the line from your ear sits in front of your shoulder, you have forward head posture.

To resolve forward head posture, do the Head, Neck, and Upper Back Routine (page 75).

You may find that in the picture you have forward head posture (FHP), but with the wall test, you can touch the back of your head to the wall. This means that you have a correctible forward head posture. Some people who have had serious postural issues for years may have what is known as a fixed posture. This happens when the forward head posture has been maintained for such a long time that the tissues have become less pliable, or the vertebral bodies and discs actually change shape because of the continuous force.

Of course, there are other causes of forward head posture, such as congenital changes of the shape of the vertebral bodies (Scheuermann's kyphosis, Klippel-Feil syndrome); post-traumatic changes to the shape of a vertebra after a fracture or infection; and changes associated with inflammatory arthritis. If you have any of these conditions, you could still benefit from trying to restore your Foundation for Movement, but your expectations may have to change regarding your ability to improve the overall alignment of your head and neck. If you are one of the few who have severe structural changes in your upper thoracic spine or neck, it makes it harder (in some cases impossible) to correct a fixed FHP deformity. You may be literally stuck in a forward head posture. So, you may ask, *Why bother doing any exercises if I cannot fix the alignment pillar?* Well, there are a couple of good reasons. Doing the exercises can prevent your posture from progressively getting worse. This is key. Not only is pain an issue with FHP, there are other health effects such as decreased lung capacity (hard to take in a deep breath), digestive disorders (when the chest collapses onto the abdomen, it affects the internal organs), and poor balance. Importantly, most of my patients report decreased pain with improved muscle activation to support their fixed forward head position; even a few degrees of improvement and better muscular support for your upper back and neck can do wonders.

Rarely Too Late

If I had completely ignored everything that I know about a Foundation for Movement, my neck might have become more like my patient Paulie's. Paulie was a publishing executive, and after retiring from a life of manuscripts, Paulie had gone back to school at Columbia University to study social work. As an editor and a social worker, Paulie read a lot of books. More than anyone I've ever met. The problem is that Paulie, like most people, sits when he reads, and all that sitting has consequences. The effect of gravity on a 10-pound head—or a 12-pound head if you've got a brain as big as Paulie's—creates serious postural imbalances.

At first, Paulie's neck pain lasted only an hour or two. Then he started waking up in the morning with a crick in his neck. First, he blamed his pillow. Later, those cricks turned into cracks that sounded like a haunted house. Ten years after it first began, the pain was almost unbearable. His arm was often numb and uncomfortable.

When Paulie went to his family doctor, he was told that all his nerves were working, but he had a bit of arthritis in his neck. He was prescribed analgesics and massage. The massages did make him feel much better—but only for a day or two. The problem, an X-ray revealed, was moderate to severe degenerative disc disease in the cervical spine, most intensely at the C5/C6 level on the right, the most commonly affected area related to age. The massages eased the pain because they relaxed the muscles around his arthritic spine, but they did nothing to address the root causes—the forces across his neck—and so the symptoms came right back shortly after treatment.

Following an MRI of his neck, Paulie was told that he had moderate disc herniations. There was narrowing of the neural foramen (the tunnel through which the nerves exit the spinal canal), but fortunately there was no pressure on the spinal cord itself. Despite Paulie's symptoms of weakness and numbness, when the nerves were tested, everything worked.

Paulie, like most of my patients, grew very worried after learning the MRI reported a disc herniation. People immediately believe that they need surgery. This is not always the case, and more often than not, surgery is *not* required. I told Paulie what I tell everyone: "You have to change the way you move." Paulie needed to address the foundational concerns, as I had done, with the big difference being how quickly his tissues would respond. Once there are structural changes, like a loss of disc height, it becomes more difficult to restore your spine to normal, but this does not mean we should not try.

Look Deeper

Even if you are experiencing shoulder or elbow pain, you may want to consider FHP as the culprit. I once worked with Brett, a pitcher at the highest level of junior league baseball in America, dreaming of college scholarships and the big leagues. There was just one problem: elbow pain. Fearing he'd lose his spot on the team, Brett didn't say anything—until one day when it was impossible not to.

After tossing 100 balls in a single game, Brett's forearm felt really tight. He often felt fatigue in his throwing arm, but this was different. Soon the tightness evolved, and he developed pain on the inside of his elbow. His pitches started slowing, and his coaches began to take notice. When they questioned him, Brett finally admitted that he was in a lot of pain. His coaches put him on the disabled list and sent him to the team trainer. During Brett's assessment, the trainer noticed some loss of full extension—the inability to completely straighten the elbow—and tenderness over the tendon on the inside of the elbow and over the ligament on that same side.

With rest, Brett's elbow began to feel better. But as he started pitching again, the pain returned. X-rays and an MRI showed that while his elbow was still lacking a few degrees of extension, there was no swelling or structural problems. Under stress testing, the ligament seemed stable. However, there was one very interesting finding, one that could easily have been dismissed: tightness at the back of his right shoulder and poor positioning of the shoulder blade.

Could it be that the poor position of his shoulder blade was contributing to his elbow pain? And if it was, how did his shoulder get to be in such a position to begin with?

This all goes back to the kinetic chain, where movement at one joint affects the way another joint moves. When Brett raised his arm, he experienced a pinching feeling in the rotator cuff tendon in his shoulder. To avoid this pinching feeling, Brett altered the mechanics of his throw. After a long workout, the smaller muscles around the shoulder blade and in his back became fatigued and didn't work as well; that placed more stress on the posterior capsule (which stimulated thickening of the capsule) and required other muscles to take over. Once the shoulder mechanics were altered, the ligaments around the elbow were exposed to more stress. If he had continued to ignore the situation, ultimately the tissues would have torn completely.

Fortunately for Brett, the MRI confirmed that he had not torn the ulnar collateral ligament in his elbow, but sure enough, he had significant forward head posture with rounded thoracic spine, a tight posterior capsule in the shoulder, and weakness of the muscles that stabilize the shoulder girdle. Hence the poor position of the shoulder blade and the pinching in his rotator cuff that had unconsciously caused him to compensate and overload his elbow. This was good news, as Brett would likely respond well to a rehabilitation program. In fact, in the end, Brett got his Division I college scholarship.

People with neck issues commonly have shoulder problems and vice versa, so don't skip testing your shoulders in the next section, even if they don't appear to be the root cause of any neck pain you're experiencing. If you have lost your Foundation for Movement in one part of your body, it is likely that the areas above and below have developed compensations, so keep an eye on the adjacent body parts.

Support Your Emotions

Sometimes working to correct your movement or posture means supporting your emotions too. In Brett's case, his fear of losing the opportunity to pursue his dream got in the way of him seeking the early treatment that would have addressed his elbow pain quickly and eliminated a lot of suffering and the potential for far more serious injuries.

In my case, my bad posture might have started when I was a teenager. I grew about eight inches in two years when I was 16 years old. I went from five foot four to six feet tall and was really self-conscious about my height, a hard thing to hide. When people are calling you a giraffe, you try to shrink. It felt personal because the comments were directed at me, my height, and my perception of being feminine. I was not about to have leg shortening surgery to fit in, so I slouched in an effort to make myself seem less tall.

When I got a little older, and after a little therapy, I realized that the judgment I felt was really the other person's problem—and a societal problem too. With time, I accepted my height and the power that came with it. Height is a big advantage in certain sports, and clothes look great on a taller frame too. No matter how strong your muscles are, if you don't feel confident in yourself, it is hard to maintain healthy movements.

Some people hold stress in their trapezius muscles, which promotes a forward head posture position. Using your breath is so important to deal with not only physical but emotional pain. Visit page 192 to try the Mindful Breathing Practice, which can help relax tense muscles and give you a quiet space from those overactive emotions.

Have You Considered Your Pillow?

If you've committed to doing the exercises on the following pages regularly and you still find you wake up in the morning with a sore neck, it may be you slept so soundly with your neck in the wrong position that you accidently stressed a muscle or joint or aggravated a nerve root. This could be just a one-off, but if it is happening regularly, I would look at your pillow. There are a million pillows out there. A good pillow supports your normal neck alignment—yep, you got it, one of the pillars! Check if your head and neck are properly aligned when you are in bed; your neck should be in neutral alignment, whether you sleep on your back or side. Neutral alignment means that your head is centred in the middle of your body (lining up with your belly button), and the pillow should support the normal gentle curve of your neck. If you have the wrong pillow, your neck may be too flexed or extended, and this stresses the neck structures, which over time can create issues. It is easier, of course, if you are only a back sleeper or only a side sleeper, but if you are like me, a flipper, the height of our pillow needs to adjust to our position. A pillow positioned for proper alignment when you're on your back will not support proper alignment on your side. I use a feather pillow so that I can mould it to support my neck however I am positioned. Operate on your pillow, not on your neck!

Restoring Your Foundation for Movement

Proper posture ensures that all the right muscles are engaged and your traps aren't working alone to hold up your head. But telling yourself to sit up straight is not the answer. You might be able to do it for a couple minutes—at least that is how long I lasted before I realized I was slumped over again! This is because I did not have the right muscles activated to maintain my good alignment.

We need a multi-step approach to the problem. First, you have to loosen up the tight muscles, tendons, and fascia that hold up your head, and then you must activate the deep stabilizing muscles that have been sleeping. It becomes a positive cycle. Once all the correct muscles are working to hold up your head in proper alignment, your head only weighs 10 pounds again. When you break the cycle of tight tissue and deactivated muscles, you restore proper alignment and regain range of motion.

After your posture is corrected and all the right muscles are engaged, your traps will no longer be so chronically overloaded, and your pain will start to dissipate. The right signals will be sent to your body, giving it the chance to repair, remodel, and restore normal tissue quality and balance. This is an amazing process. We can direct and control how our body breaks down or heals depending on how we move. I prescribe the exercises in a specific order, starting with the release of tight tissues, usually with ASMR, and then always following up with an activation through a full range of motion to solidify a new movement pattern and remodel the body.

CORRECTING LONG-STANDING IMBALANCES

If the imbalance is fairly new, changing your movement is usually enough for your body to remodel the tissue and correct the imbalance. It never ceases to amaze me how quickly imbalances correct themselves and pain dissipates when we use the right muscles. However, if an imbalance has developed over years, the tissue will have restructured, becoming so stiff you'll need to lengthen and soften it first. The first goal is to improve tissue pliability.

Think of a tree in the wind. When this tree is first exposed to wind, it moves in the direction it is blown, but once the wind stops, the flexible branch can return to its usual position. Now imagine the tree has spent 20 years with the wind blowing in one direction. With the constant stress of the wind, the branches have changed their growth pattern in response. Even when the wind stops blowing, the tree's wind-blown shape is maintained.

Our body is similar: Tissue loses its pliability because of long-standing imbalances. However, when we stretch or stimulate the area—be it through massage, acupuncture, physiotherapy, laser therapy, foam rolling, or, ideally, active stretching (when a muscle pulls on the tissue)—we increase blood supply to the region, hydrating the tissue. Once the tissues are hydrated and pliable, they can then begin to work normally and become more balanced. But it takes time for permanent changes in the tissue to occur.

Foam rolling and active self-myofascial release are great tools to improve tissue pliability. Many of the exercises we teach use a tool such as a foam roller or a massage ball to apply pressure to tissue. Think of rolling out pie dough: You apply pressure to the dough, and it changes shape. We don't flatten out our tissues to the same degree, but the rolling changes the tissues at a molecular level, improving hydration and stimulating them to bind more water.

Active self-myofascial release is a technique that we use to loosen muscles, tendons, or fascia that are adherent, or stuck, to surrounding connective tissues; that prevents gliding, hinders muscle activation, and limits joint range of motion. The Head, Neck, and Upper Back Routine starts by releasing a muscle that is commonly tight and does not move well, the upper trapezius. The upper traps sits on the side of your neck and top of your shoulder. If you place your hand on the left side of your neck and touch your ear to your right shoulder, you will feel the upper trapezius pop up into your hand. From the traps, we move on to the supine chin tuck (discussed in detail later) to activate some of the deep muscles in our neck that are not commonly used.

As I worked to improve my neck posture, I made sure that I also improved the position of the operating room table so that I could maintain my posture properly while I worked, and I got a pair of glasses. If you are suffering from neck pain, headaches, and forward head posture, think about your workstation, your driving posture, and how you can adjust your head and neck position during activities that last for a prolonged period of time. Sometimes you cannot adjust your environment, and that makes it even more important to build up your Foundation for Movement. Build endurance and strength in the muscles of your neck and shoulder girdles to manage the extra stress. Take frequent breaks to reset your foundation, and ensure that the deep stabilizing muscles are working even though your neck may not be in an optimal position.

TROUBLESHOOTING AND COMMON STUMBLING BLOCKS

The neck is a challenging area of the body to manage as there are a lot of important structures travelling from the brain to the body. The main reason we have a neck is to position our sensory organs—our eyes, our ears, and our nose—so that we can see, hear, and smell our surroundings. The muscles in our neck are unique: They have more proprioceptors than other muscles, meaning they have an important role in maintaining balance. Major blood vessels and nerves enter and exit various pathways in the neck. So, changes in the position and structure of our neck can affect many different systems. Below are some common issues that I encounter in my clinical practice. Be aware of them before you start your new exercise routine, and don't be discouraged if your progress isn't as quick as you'd like.

- If you spend 15 to 30 minutes a day doing these exercises, but then sit in your car, at a desk, or stand in the operating room all day with bad posture, it will take longer to improve. Check out Chapter 11 for some tips to correct old habits. Do an ergonomic assessment of your workstation, check your posture in your car and the position of your mirrors, get that new pillow, and set an alarm for a posture check throughout the day. As you get stronger and are activating the right muscles, you will naturally hold your posture more effortlessly. Give yourself time.
- Many people get a headache the first few days of performing the routine. With all the changes to the muscles and fascia, sensory nerves can get temporarily aggravated. It is likely that the tissues in your neck have been short for a *long*, *long* time. Give it a few days, and as the tissues remodel and adjust, the headache will go away. Go slowly, apply a little heat after exercise and before bed, and don't force anything.

- For those with significant FHP—either fixed or extreme posture so that you cannot touch your head to the wall when you stand up straight—you need to realize that you will make tiny changes and progress will be slow. Let your body adjust to the new exercises, and slowly, over six months, nine months, a year, it will improve. It probably took over a decade for the forward head posture to develop, so be patient.
- Do you hear cracking noises or feel grinding sensations when doing the exercises? I don't fuss about these unless they are really painful. The majority of the time, these sensations are not painful, and the intensity of the noise usually lessens with time. The noise could be caused by some fascia or a ligament starting to remodel or by a small joint cracking. If the crack is really painful, stop what you are doing and re-evaluate. If the symptoms persist or are associated with any of the red flag symptoms, follow up as directed below.
- Watch out for these red flag symptoms: If you experience numbness, tingling, weakness, bowel or bladder changes, or significant pain radiating down your arm, you should get a checkup with your family doctor. In the vast majority of cases, everything is fine, and once you are cleared, you can use the symptom as feedback. For example, if you are doing an exercise and you get increased numbness in your arm, back off the intensity and observe yourself doing the movement. Better yet, have a therapist observe you to ensure you are using proper form. The goal is to gradually ease into the contraction and stay at the intensity where you have no symptoms or pain less than 3 on the NPRS. If you have pain with movement, decrease the amount of movement to the pain-free range. Often when we start an exercise program, our tight fascia, muscles, and nerves do not glide well, but as you slowly move the tissues with the exercises, your symptoms will resolve.

Head, Neck, and Upper Back Routine

The conventional approach to pain in the neck is to stretch the muscles that feel achy and tense. However, this approach only addresses the symptoms, not the root causes. The Head, Neck, and Upper Back Routine will help you achieve symptom relief *and* gets to the root causes to restore pain-free neck movement and mobility that lasts.

The first time you perform any new exercise, focus primarily on following the technique cues given. Don't worry so much about counting reps. Once you feel you have a basic grasp of the exercise, start your first set slow and gradually increase how hard you contract your muscles. Work toward increasing your range of motion for the exercise. Rest for 30 to 60 seconds between each set and between exercises.

IF YOU DON'T HAVE NECK PAIN: Cycle through the Head, Neck, and Upper Back Routine along with the other routines according to the Movement Longevity Schedule (page 196) that best accommodates your lifestyle.

IF YOU DO HAVE NECK PAIN: Alternate the Head, Neck, and Upper Back Routine with the Shoulder and Arm Routine (page 101) daily for four weeks. You can take one day off each week if you so choose. You should notice a significant decrease or complete elimination of pain. Continue with a Movement Longevity Schedule (page 196). If your NPRS rating is greater than or equal to 7, do the Head, Neck, and Upper Back Routine for Acute Pain (page 87).

Lateral Neck Active Self-Myofascial Release

Relieves muscular tension and knots and restores length to the neck muscles that often tense up from pain and stress.

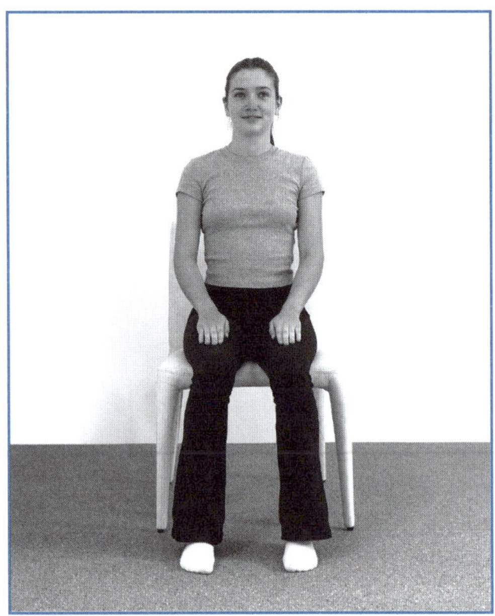

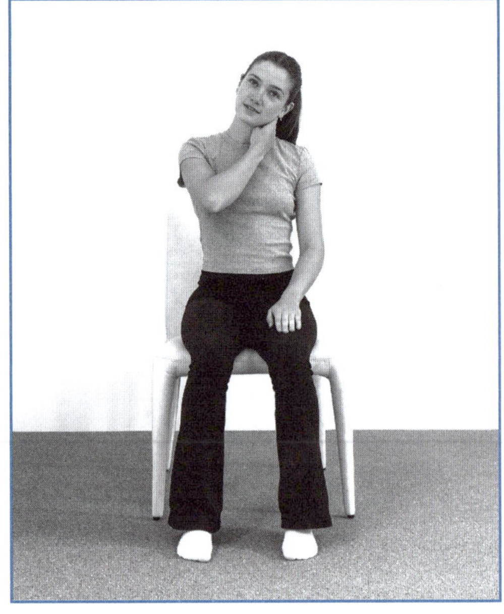

1. Sit or stand comfortably in good posture, with your shoulders slightly back and your head and upper back straight and tall, as if there's a string attached to the top of your head pulling you straight up.
2. Tilt your head to the left so your left ear moves toward your left shoulder.
3. Press the fingers of your right hand into the muscles on the left side of your neck just below your ear as much as you can tolerate without excessive pain.
4. Relax your muscles as much as possible so your fingers can dig in.

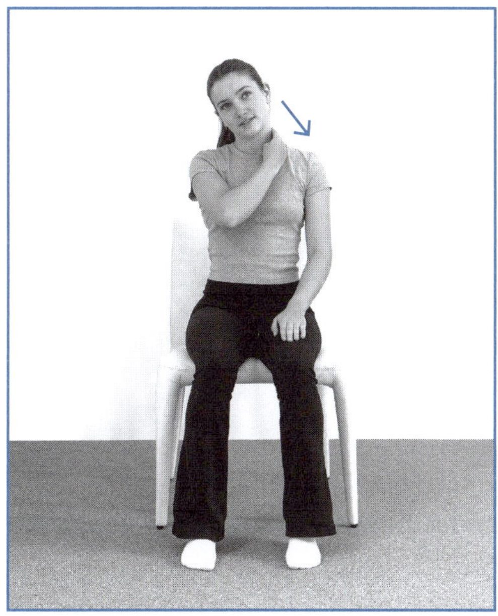

5. Slowly tilt your head in the opposite direction as you simultaneously slide your fingers down your neck toward your collarbone.
6. Work your fingers in different areas of the muscle.
7. Continue for one minute on each side.

Segmental Cat-Camel

Restores segmental movement through the whole spine and activates the deep muscles that contribute to stability and posture.

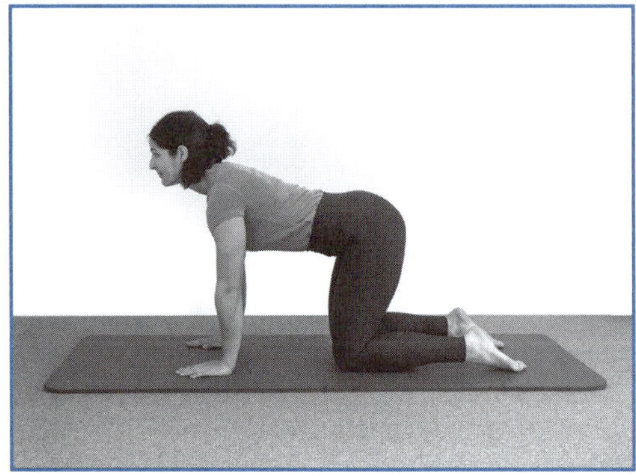

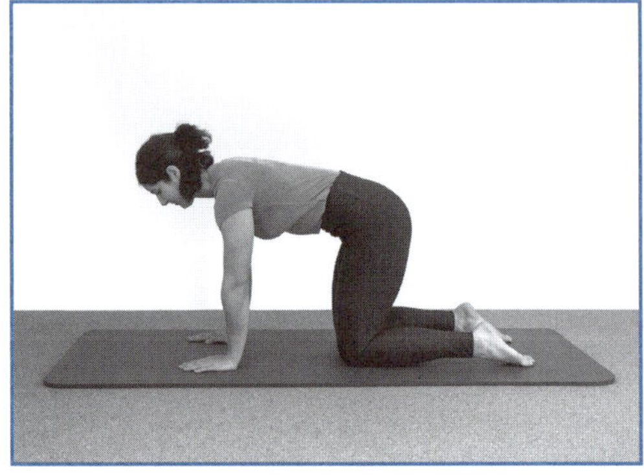

1. Start with your hands and knees on the ground with your back arched and head up looking straight ahead.
2. Tilt your pelvis down as if you have a tail and you're tucking it between your legs.

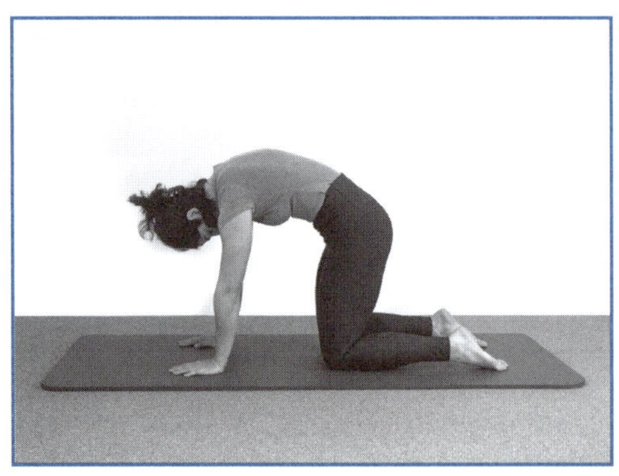

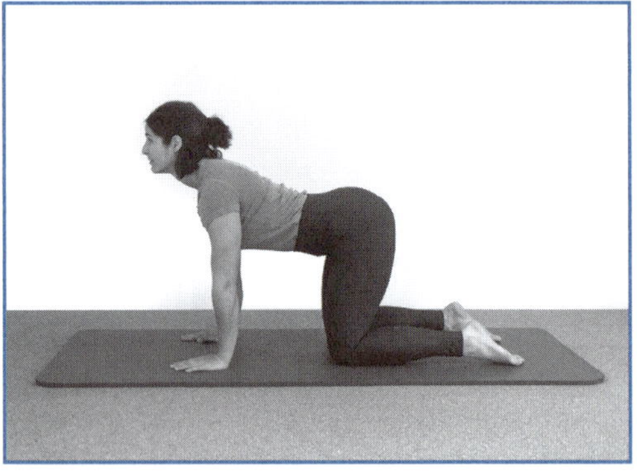

3. From the bottom up, round the spine about an inch at a time until your back is fully curved like a C and you're looking at your knees.
4. Tilt your pelvis up as if you were putting your tail into the air.

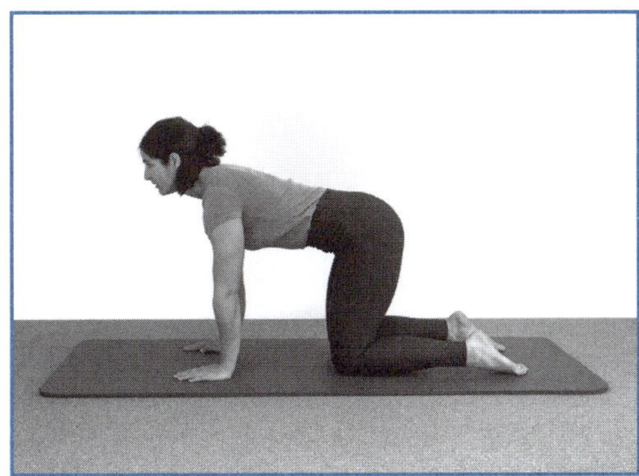

5. From the bottom up, extend the spine about an inch at a time until you return to the starting position with your head up and looking straight ahead.
6. Repeat steps 1 through 5 six times.

Segmental Thoracic Mob

Improves posture and function by increasing movement of the joints in the upper and middle back while waking up the muscles that contribute to both mobility and stability.

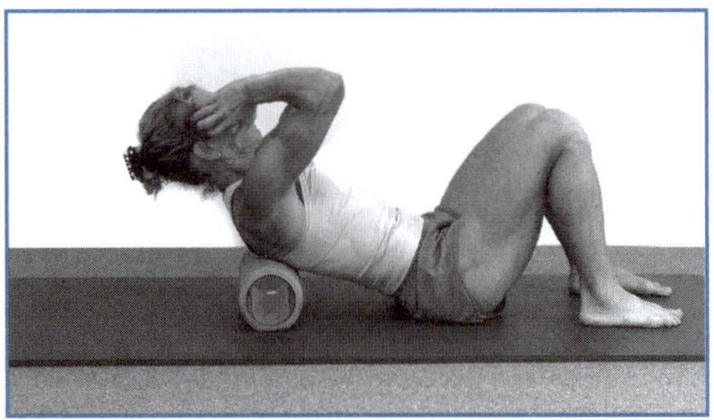

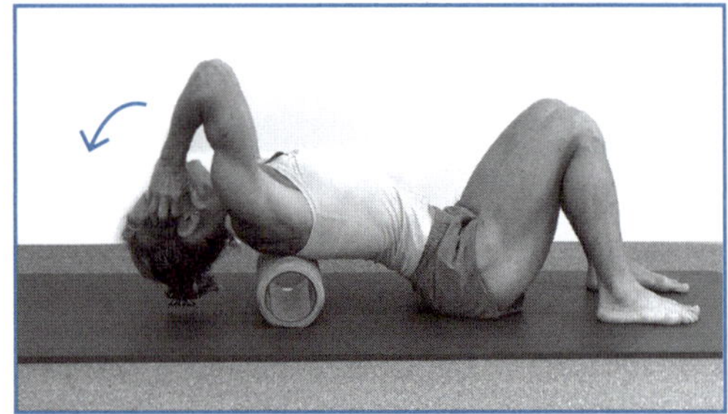

1. Lie over a standard foam roller or a yoga block with the support object at the bottom of your shoulder blades. Place your hands at your temples or gently hold your head in a neutral position if you need extra support. If lying down over the roller strains your neck or is otherwise too uncomfortable, you can perform the exercise standing with the roller between your back and the wall.
2. Extend your upper back over the support object, bringing your head as close to the floor as possible, then return to neutral. Repeat three times.

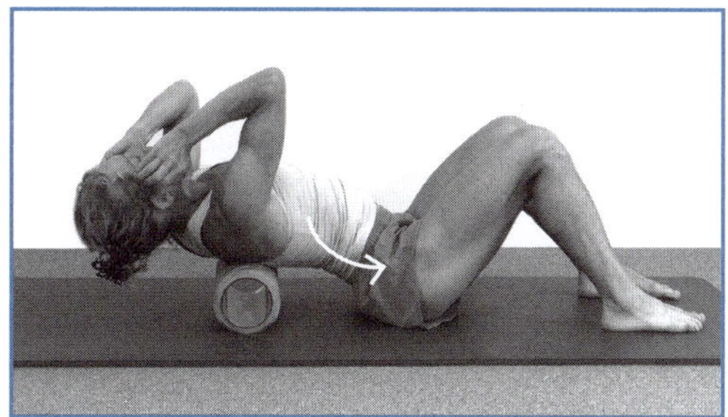

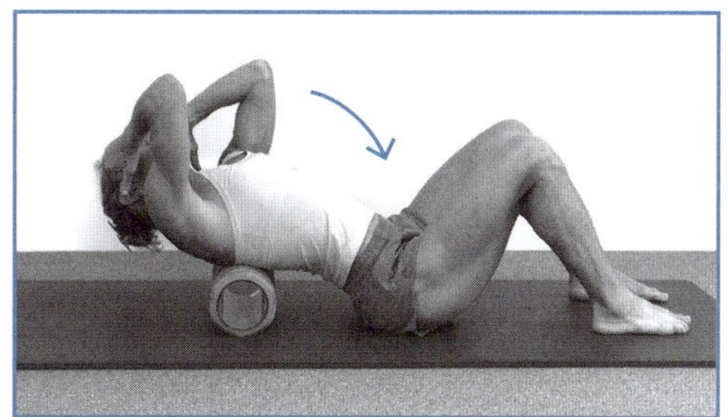

3. With your body extended over the support object, side bend, bringing armpit to hip. Repeat three times on each side.

4. With your body extended over the support object, rotate through your upper spine to look from one side to the other for three reps on each side.

5. Move the support object about one inch closer to your neck. Repeat steps 2 to 4 in the new position.

6. Continue until you've worked four to five segments up toward the base of your neck.

Six-Way Neck Isometric

Activates the stabilizer muscles of the neck, which can provide some rapid pain relief, and solidifies good posture.

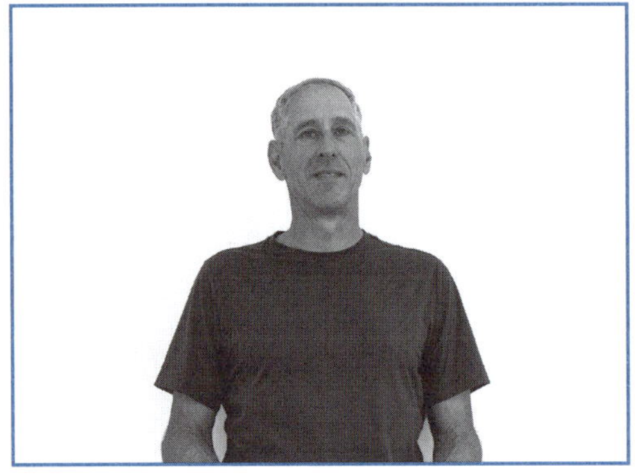

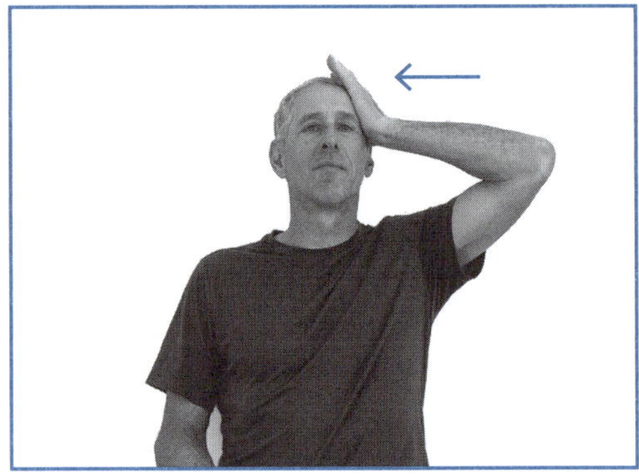

1. For each of the following six positions, sit or stand in good posture. Gradually increase the amount of pressure you apply to your head (as long as you're not feeling pain). Breathe naturally.
2. Press your left hand into the left side of your head just above your ear. Hold for five seconds.

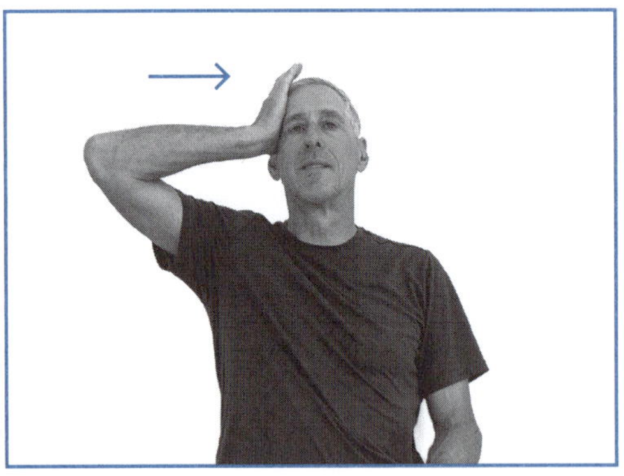

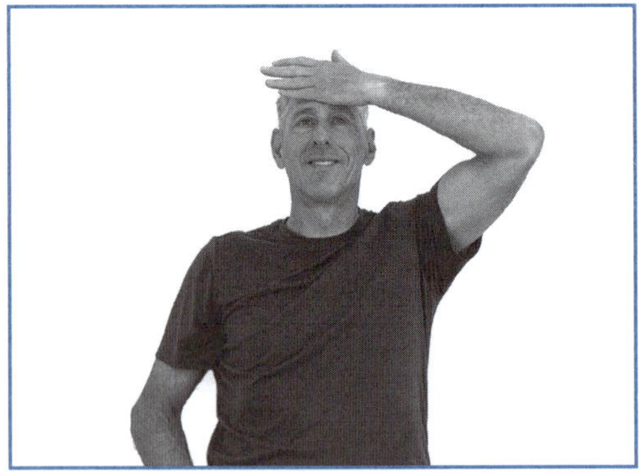

3. Repeat with your right hand pressing on the right side of your head.
4. Press your left hand into your forehead. Hold for five seconds.

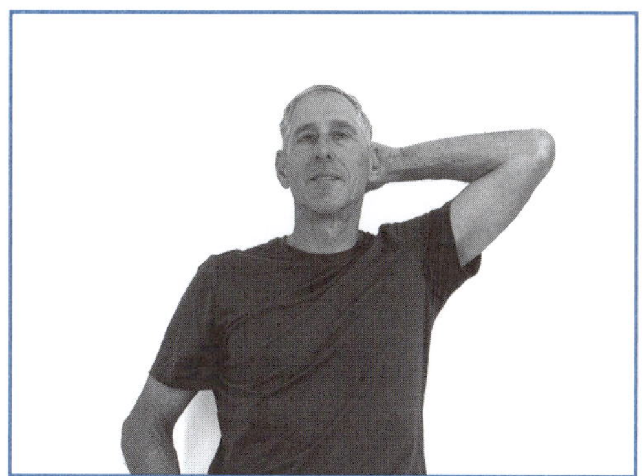

5. Press your right hand into the back of your head. Hold for five seconds.

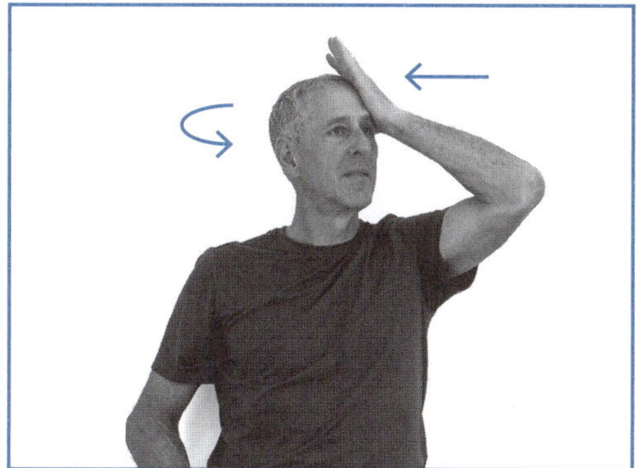

6. Press your left hand into the left side of your head near your temple, and try to rotate your head to the left. Hold for five seconds.

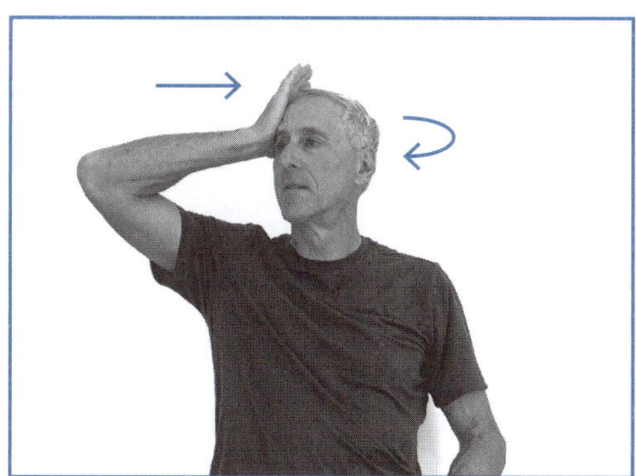

7. Press your right hand into the right side of your head near your temple, and try to rotate your head to the right. Hold for five seconds.

8. Repeat steps 1 to 7 three times.

Forward Head and Scapula Elevation Dissociation

Breaks the common associated movement pattern of shrugging the shoulders that results in a forward head position, thus helping to restore good posture for the long term.

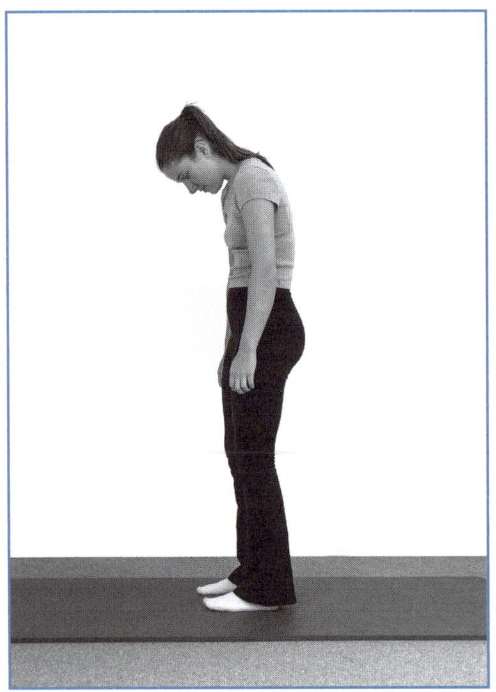

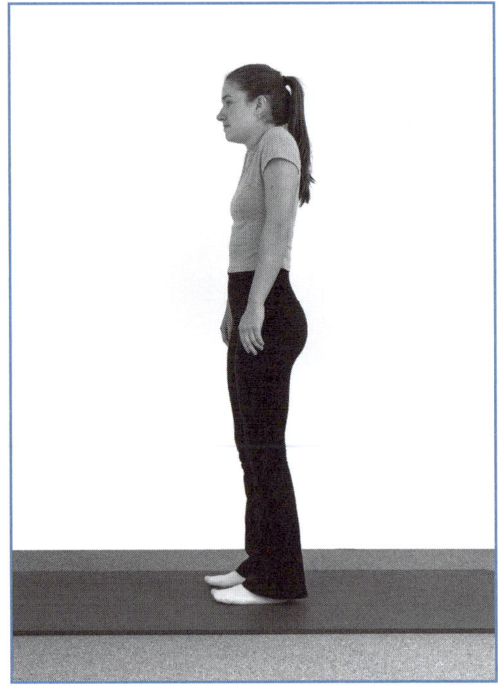

1. Stand and round your spine into poor posture with your head jutting forward and your mid- and upper back rounded, so your body is in a C shape. Gently pull your shoulders down towards your hips.
2. Shrug your shoulders as you stand up into good posture, and hold for 5 seconds while breathing naturally.
3. Return to the starting position, and repeat eight times.

Wall Neck Side Bend

Relaxes the often-tense muscles on the side of your neck, like the upper trapezius and levator scapulae, while simultaneously strengthening and lengthening them.

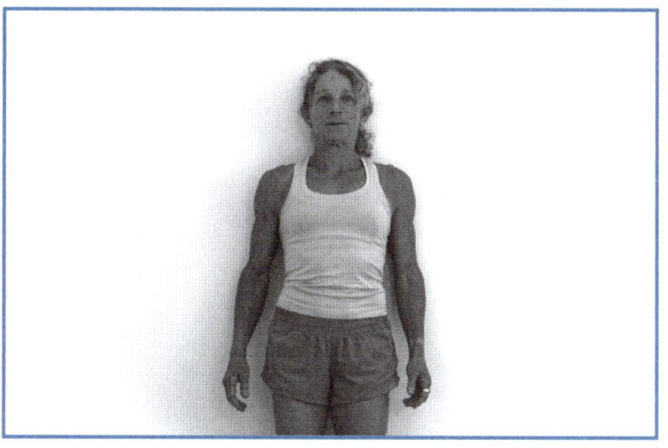

1. Stand with good posture with your head and back against a wall and your heels about six inches away from the wall. If you cannot touch your head to the wall, get as close as possible.

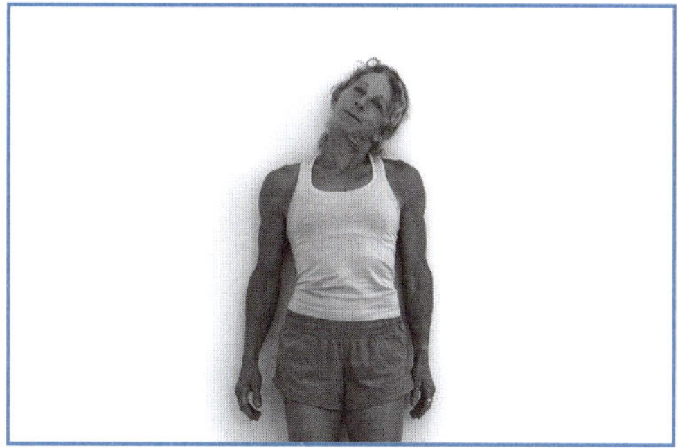

2. Inhale and then slowly exhale while bringing your left ear toward your left shoulder as far as you can without pain. Hold for two seconds.
3. Exhale and bring your neck back to a neutral position.

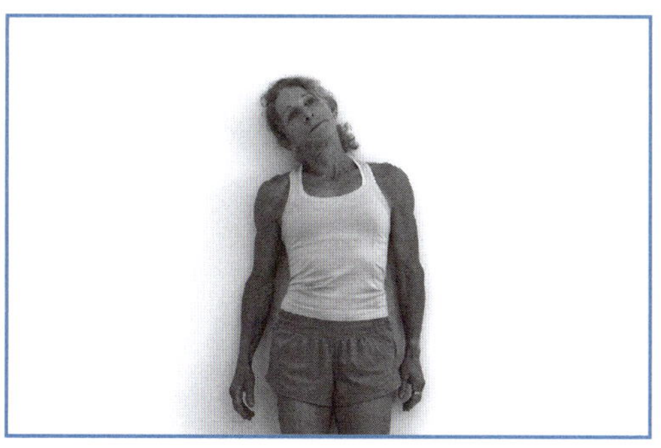

4. Inhale and then slowly exhale while bringing your right ear toward your right shoulder as far as you can without pain. Hold for two seconds.

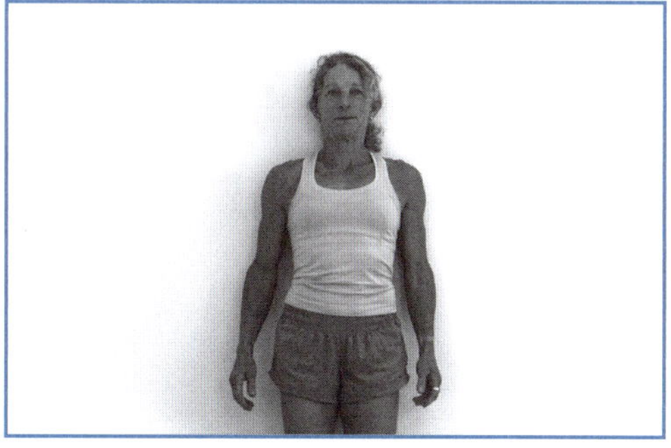

5. Exhale and bring your neck back to a neutral position.
6. Repeat steps 2 through 5 eight times.

Supine Chin Tuck

Lengthens the upper spine and activates the deep cervical neck flexor muscles, which are critical for neck stability and good posture.

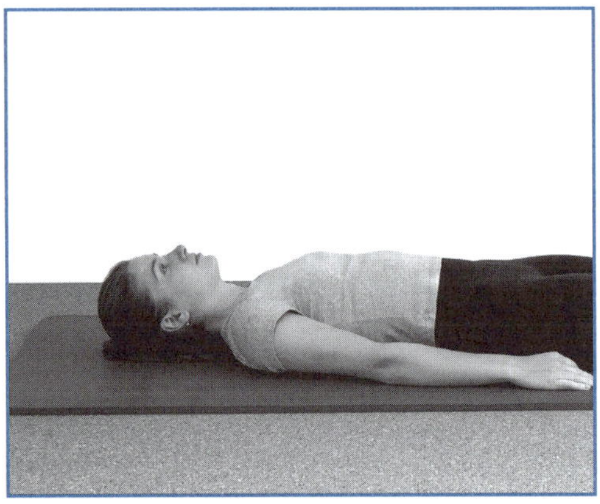

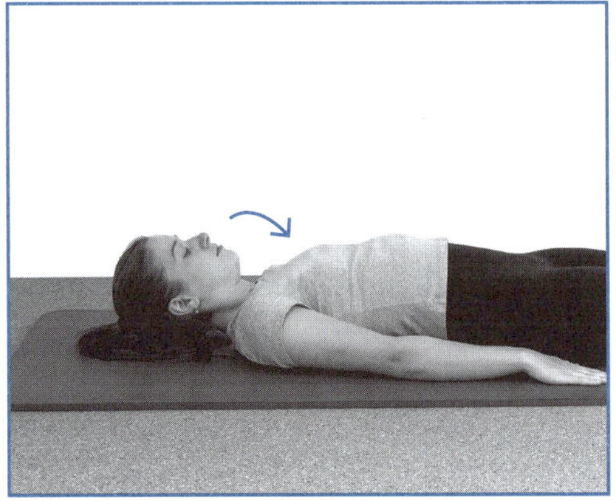

1. Lie down on the floor with your shoulder blades pinched together slightly. If you cannot lie with your head resting comfortably on the floor, you can use a pillow that is just high enough so that your spine remains neutral and you aren't straining your neck.
2. Draw your chin in toward the floor while imagining there is a string pulling your head backwards to lengthen your spine. Hold for one breath or about five seconds.
3. Keeping your chin tucked, lift your head off the ground just enough that a piece of paper could be slid underneath. Hold for five seconds.
4. Gently lower your head back to floor, and release the chin tuck.
5. Repeat steps 2 through 4 ten times.

Head, Neck, and Upper Back Routine for Acute Pain

If you are in pain greater than or equal to a 7 on the NPRS, do this Head, Neck, and Upper Back Routine for Acute Pain to bring down your pain. Complete this routine in the morning after you get up, at lunchtime, dinnertime, and again before bed. It will help settle your symptoms so that you can start the standard Head, Neck, and Upper Back Routine described above.

Lateral Neck Active Self-Myofascial Release *(pages 76–77)*

Relieves muscular tension and knots and restores length to the neck muscles that often tense up from pain and stress.

Six-Way Neck Isometric *(pages 82–83)*

Activates the stabilizer muscles of the neck, which can provide some rapid pain relief, and solidifies good posture.

CHAPTER 6

Shoulders and Arms

During my residency training, I was working so hard that I did not have time to play sports, which had been a big part of my life. I got exercise by running to the hospital each morning. I would leave home at around 5 a.m.; at work, I had to round on 30 patients before attending teaching rounds at 7 a.m., followed by the OR at 8 a.m.; then we had to prepare our patients for the operating room for the next day before heading home or staying the night to cover the emergency room. Needless to say, I did not do any warm-up or cool-down. Now I know this pace and workload are a recipe for losing one's Foundation for Movement.

Once I entered my surgical practice and was in charge of my own schedule (or so I thought), I began to play tennis. Initially, I played once a week with my friend Diana, but I had been bitten badly by the tennis bug and I hated that she would beat me 6–1. (She is very gracious and always gave me one game.) I do not like losing and wanted to improve, so I started taking lessons. It was around this time that I noticed my posture was not ideal and my shoulders were really rounded.

One evening while brushing my teeth, I looked in the mirror and noticed that my right shoulder was much lower than my left. This is something that I have seen for years with my patients, particularly overhead athletes, like pitchers, and anyone who has done repetitive movements with their upper extremity, including painters and assembly line workers. I was surprised to see how out of balance my right shoulder was. In my case, the shoulder imbalances were related to how I was positioned when working in the operating room, as well as my younger years as an athlete playing volleyball, tennis, basketball, track and field, downhill skiing, and softball. It was all compounded by increasing my tennis workouts.

So, how exactly did my shoulder get so low? To fully understand why a part of the body breaks down, it is important to understand the function of the connective tissues around the shoulder.

What Makes a Healthy Shoulder

The shoulder is a variation of a ball and socket joint; in this case, the socket is more like a saucer, which allows for greater range of motion than the deep socket of the hip joint. The rotator cuff (supraspinatus tendon), a common site of injury, is a collection of muscles and tendons (the subscapularis, supraspinatus, infraspinatus, and teres minor) whose job is to stabilize the shoulder. It's the rotator cuff's job to keep the ball of the humerus bone centred on the saucer, which is called the glenoid. If it's able to do its job, the joint is less likely to get injured. Just like a car that is in danger of wearing out a tire if out of alignment, the shoulder structures are at risk of breaking down if not properly aligned.

Any time you move your arm, you're using the tendons and muscles of the rotator cuff to keep your shoulder aligned. Of the four tendons in the rotator cuff, the supraspinatus is the most vulnerable and usually the first to tear because it has a poor blood supply; when our alignment is off, it is susceptible to mechanical impingement (pinching of the tendon).

The shoulder blade, the mobile platform where the glenohumeral joint is based, often becomes poorly positioned, which leads to increased stress on the rotator cuff. This happens because of poor posture (remember I had forward head posture, see page 65), development of bone spurs, variations of normal bone anatomy (which decrease the amount of space for the tendon), repetitive motion, hand dominance, blood supply, and genetics. The first step in addressing any shoulder issue is to recognize this poor placement: The position of the shoulder blade must be corrected to fully recover from a rotator cuff overload.

When we perform a repetitive movement, such as throwing a fastball or hammering on the job, our arm must move quickly to propel the ball or hammer, and once the action is completed, the muscles at the back of the shoulder must slow our arm to its normal resting position. If the muscles of deceleration (slowing down the body) become fatigued, the shoulder blade's natural position is compromised. And if there's repetitive force applied to the connective tissues at the back of the shoulder, the body responds by reinforcing (and thickening) the tissue. This seems like a sensible response, but thicker fascia changes how the entire joint moves. Instead of the humerus staying centred on the glenoid when you lift your arm overhead, the humeral head gets pushed upward. Because of this, the supraspinatus tendon gets pushed up into a bony part of the shoulder blade, which impinges and shuts off the muscle in turn. This is the start of a vicious cycle: Tight posterior connective tissue leads to increased rotator cuff impingement, which weakens the rotator cuff, leading to more impingement, pain, and, after many years, a tendon tear.

DO YOU LACK A STRONG FOUNDATION IN YOUR SHOULDERS?

1. Standing up straight, reach one arm up and over your head, while resting your opposite hand by your side. Turn your palm to face your back, and reach down between your shoulder blades as far as you can. Hold this position. Using your opposite hand with your palm facing out, reach for your other hand from below. Try to touch your hands together. If you can touch, you pass the test, which means your shoulder foundation is solid. If not, ask a buddy to measure the distance between your fingers. This will give you a benchmark so you can measure your progress after doing the exercises below. Those with hypermobility (super-flexible joints) should be mindful not to stick out their chest and abdomen to make their hands connect. For the best assessment, your chest and abdomen should remain in a neutral position.

2. Repeat the test, raising the opposite arm overhead. It is very common to fail this test when your dominant side is reaching from below. The goal is to be able to touch your fingers to one another regardless of which arm is overhead, or at least decrease the distance between them over time.

If you lack a foundation in your shoulders, do the Shoulder and Arm Routine (page 101).

Don't forget: The body is connected from head to toe, so imbalances in other parts of the body will affect the shoulder. The most common postural imbalance I see today that affects the shoulder is forward head posture, which we discussed in the previous chapter (page 65). Many of the muscles that control neck function connect to the scapula (shoulder blade), so you can imagine how tightness or weakness in these muscles intimately affects the position and movement of the shoulder platform, which then leads to abnormal scapular positioning, decreasing the space for the rotator cuff tendons to glide and making them more vulnerable to impingement.

Further Challenges from Repetitive Motion

Repetitive movements of the arm can also create increased mechanical stress, and tiny outgrowths of bone called spurs may develop, which further decrease space for the tendon. When the tendon gets pinched due to bone spurs, the rotator cuff tendons start to wear and you'll experience mechanical impingement. Much like your car keys distressing the pocket of your jeans, this is harmless at first. But over time, a hole develops. How quickly a hole develops in the rotator cuff tendon depends partly upon the intensity and duration of your movements. Non-athletes with abnormal posture may not experience deterioration in their rotator cuff tendons for decades, but low-intensity stress over a long period of time can create a tendon tear. People who perform repetitive overhead actions—like bricklayers, baseball pitchers, tennis players, or butchers, to name a few—and endure consistent high-intensity stress may become symptomatic sooner, even in their 20s or 30s. The culprits in both situations—that is, high-intensity short-duration activities or low-intensity long-duration activities—are soft tissue imbalances, which put abnormal stress on the tendon.

In my case, I had pain when serving the tennis ball and hitting high forehands. I also got to the point where I had some pain if I lay on my right side. Even cleaning the kitchen sink was painful. There was some tendinosis and maybe a small partial tendon tear that was one or two millimetres long. But the pain was a clear indication I was stressing the tissue, and my rhythm for recovery was not ideal.

To correct my shoulder pain, I had to perform the Head, Neck, and Upper Back Routine (page 75) and the Shoulder and Arm Routine (page 101) to adequately create a Foundation for Movement for my neck and shoulder girdle. My symptoms quickly resolved over a couple of weeks. Like me, most people with shoulder problems have issues with their neck and therefore I always recommend doing both programs. Because we have to reprogram the muscles around both the spine and the shoulder blade to create the proper platform for the rotator cuff to work, dissociation techniques are emphasized in these routines. As always, I recommend releasing the tight structures first, before activating and reprogramming the muscles.

Never Too Late

As long as a connection between the tendon tissue in your shoulder exists, your body is capable of repairing the area. If an ultrasound or MRI reports tendinosis or a tiny (1–2 millimetres) partial tear of the tendon in your shoulder, you can start to repair your body by changing how you move. If, however, you change how you move but the activity you want to do is too strenuous, then you may end up like my dear friend and tennis doubles partner, Abbi. We were playing together in a national tournament when I noticed that her shoulder was bothering her. It especially hurt when she served or hit an overhead ball or a high backhand volley. Prior to this tournament, her pain would recede with rest, but it always came right back as soon as she started playing again.

I took a look at Abbi's shoulder, and sure enough, she had all the hallmarks of an overhead athlete: a tight posterior capsule, a weak rotator cuff, and a shoulder blade lowered and tilted toward the front. I gave her a list of exercises much like the ones in our program, and she did them diligently. Soon her shoulder began to improve, and she noticed a big difference in her day-to-day life, but she still couldn't play tennis. It just hurt too much.

An MRI revealed that Abbi had a significant partial tear of the supraspinatus tendon, not just a couple of millimetres but close to 80 percent of the tendon thickness. She tried playing again, but I could see that her shoulder was weak. The demands of the game were too much for the injured tendon. In her case, I knew that if she wanted to remain a serious competitor, she would need surgery. Of course, she had a choice; she could easily have chosen not to play. Her everyday life was largely unaffected, especially after finishing the exercise program I prescribed. But for Abbi, who loves tennis like I do, giving up her sport wasn't an option.

Abbi approached her surgical recovery with the same discipline she applied to training. She did pendulum swings and rotator cuff isometrics to prevent stiffness. She activated her core and its connection to the shoulder blade, and she strengthened her shoulder girdle. She did this all very carefully under the guidance of her surgeon, knowing that post-surgery recovery is incredibly delicate. The time that Abbi spent on establishing her Foundation for Movement prior to surgery kickstarted her road to recovery because she had started to address the root movement cause of her tendon tear. The trick to getting a good surgical result is to change how you're loading the rotator cuff tendon after its repair. You need to understand why the rotator cuff developed a tear so the repaired tendon doesn't suffer the same fate. It may take 9 to 12 months for the muscles to become strong enough to participate in strenuous activities.

A year after her surgery, Abbi and I won a bronze medal at the 55-plus USTA National Clay Court Championships. Next year, we're going for gold. It is great to know that you can recover from painful situations and return to high-level activity, but it is important to try to catch your problem as early as possible to give your body the chance to heal.

Going Deeper

What would have happened if Abbi had ignored her shoulder symptoms completely? Unfortunately, it's something I see a lot. In some cases, the tear slowly sneaks up over decades of unconsciously compensating for the injury. In other cases, people experience intermittent shoulder pain and get lost on a path for recovery. Too often, people just don't know what to do. They want to do something, and they think they have done something—they have rested, had cortisone injections, taken pills, and maybe even tried some exercises—but as soon as they try to return to what they love to do, which is often a significant cause of their pain, the pain rears its ugly head again, and there can be a slow progression in the wear and tear process.

Just because you have a rotator cuff tear does not mean that you must have surgery. Many people who have no symptoms and enjoy their quality of life decide not to have surgery. While others, like Abbi, opt for surgery because it's a priority for them to keep doing something they love. Even if your MRI shows that you have a torn tendon, you are not doomed for surgery.

Once we reach the tender age of 60 years, up to 40 percent of the general population will have an asymptomatic rotator cuff tendon tear. Not all tears are created equal. A two-millimetre partial thickness tear is very different from a three-centimetre full thickness tear, which again is very different from a one-centimetre full thickness tear. Despite the differences, doctors typically refer to each of these scenarios as a rotator cuff tendon tear! Confusing, huh? What's important to understand is what will happen to your body if you don't correct the root cause of the wear and tear problem.

In the case of a rotator cuff tear, if you ignore the pain and don't change how you move, the tear can become progressively bigger over time and eventually affect more of the tendons around the shoulder. In a worst-case scenario, you would not be able to lift your arm overhead after the tendon tears grow so big that they can no longer be repaired. Still, if you don't want to have surgery, you may not have to. You might have to make some lifestyle changes—some changes to your movement patterns. You may not be able to swing a hammer to fix your roof, but you may be able to get to a point where you can brush your hair, easily grab a glass off the top shelf of the kitchen cupboard, and perform most day-to-day tasks. If your shoulder only hurts when you do one activity, you may choose to give up that activity. Enjoying the quality of your life is what counts.

So how do you know if your rotator cuff tear is worsening? Most people who have significant pathology (tendon damage) will have some aching or notice that they have to modify the way they move. If you have a tear, I recommend keeping an eye on the size of it by getting an ultrasound every year. You can check in with your doctor to assess the size of the tear, and the doctor can also look at your Foundation for Movement.

If you have a rotator cuff tear, you *will* have to do some form of maintenance for your shoulder for your lifetime, whether you have surgery or not. At first, the exercises may be daily, but eventually it becomes two to three days per week. It all depends on how active you are, how strong your shoulder is, and how well you compensate and prevent overloading of the remaining rotator cuff tendons. Regardless of whether you have tendinosis, a partial tear, or a complete tear of the tendon, the exercise solution is the same. It will just take a little longer to restore your foundation if you have a full thickness tear. The key is to obtain and maintain a Foundation for Movement to protect your tendons.

You can reach these goals by improving the biomechanics of your shoulder to take the load off the rotator cuff tear. This is achieved by addressing forward head posture, improving thoracic spine mobility, correcting the position of the scapula, and activating the scapular stabilizers as well as the rotator cuff muscles that remain intact to keep the joint properly aligned. In other words, addressing the root cause of the tendon tear by re-establishing a Foundation for Movement in the head, neck, and shoulder zones.

Don't Get Stuck Just Because Your Shoulder Is Frozen!

Active range of motion is one of the four pillars, and loss of mobility is a big impediment, particularly in the shoulder because the prime purpose a shoulder serves is to help us position our hand in space. Losing motion means a loss of function and loss of our Foundation for Movement.

Usually, a stiff shoulder is a painful shoulder. A common and challenging knock-on effect of painful wear and tear conditions affecting the shoulder is loss of mobility. When it hurts to lift an arm overhead, most of us tend to stop doing it. As a result, the tissues start to lose their elasticity and shorten. Over time, your shoulder will get stiff and you lose motion. This is often referred to as a frozen shoulder.

The first motion we lose is usually rotation (when your elbow is tucked at your side, the ability to rotate your hand away from your body or reach behind your back), then abduction (the ability to lift your arm straight out to the side), followed by forward flexion (the ability to reach in front of your body). You may notice that you cannot reach up behind your back or even get your hand to your buttock!

One of my patients, Tonya, a 50-year-old dragon boat racer, came to my office complaining of right shoulder pain. For six months, the right-handed racer had had pain over the cap of her shoulder. The pain began insidiously but was aggravated significantly when paddling.

While preparing for the senior championships, Tonya had amped up her training, and her pain followed suit. The pain progressed from superficial pain to somewhere deep inside her shoulder joint; it also began radiating down her arm and into her hand. Soon, even lifting her arm to brush her hair was painful.

Tonya went to her family doctor, who thought she had some tendinitis in the shoulder. She was given an anti-inflammatory medication and began physiotherapy. The therapist noted restricted range of motion, particularly shoulder rotation. But when the therapist tried to manipulate and stretch the shoulder, Tonya cried out in pain—it felt like torture. Worse still, her shoulder felt like it was actually getting stiffer.

And it was. Tonya's shoulder was in constant pain, even at rest. She could barely sleep, and day-to-day activities, from showering to getting dressed in the morning, were excruciating. She tried narcotics, but they did nothing to dull the pain.

Generally, when patients are in pain at rest, it's because there's an inflammatory component to their pathology, not only a structural issue (a mechanically driven pain). A frozen shoulder is common in diabetics (we think because diabetics have imbalances from overall body inflammation), but Tonya wasn't diabetic, nor did she have a history of fractures, dislocations, or tendon tears—all potential culprits. Her frozen shoulder had no known cause; it was what we physicians refer to as idiopathic.

When I examined Tonya's shoulder, I found mild diffuse muscle wasting and severe stiffness and loss of shoulder rotation, the hallmarks of a frozen shoulder. If there is significant stiffness of your shoulder, you need an X-ray to determine if the loss of mobility is due to something like degenerative arthritis, a wear and tear issue resulting in loss of the articular cartilage of the shoulder joint. If the X-ray shows no arthritis and a good joint space, then the loss of motion is most likely due to the shoulder joint capsule shrinking and getting stiff. The good news here is that there is potential for the capsule to remodel and restore range of motion.

In my experience, a frozen shoulder is a self-limiting disorder affecting the capsule of the shoulder with three phases: (1) freezing, (2) frozen, and (3) thawing. As mysteriously as the problem comes, it goes. Understanding what stage you are in can help you to avoid unnecessarily aggravating the joint and to know when to push your range of motion and when to be patient. The pain and stiffness peak (freezing), then stabilize (frozen), and ultimately spontaneously begin to resolve (thawing). The process can take up to two years. (I know that sounds like forever for someone in pain.) If you notice that you have lost shoulder rotation, your shoulder is very irritable, and you're screaming with just the slightest wrong move, such that you cannot get any shut-eye, you are in the freezing phase of the condition. Eventually you will reach a peak in your pain and limited mobility, and you will feel like you are not getting better or worse (unless, of course, you do something you should not). This plateau signals you are in the second—or the frozen—phase. You will know that you have turned the corner into the thawing stage when your pain suddenly decreases. One day, you will wake up and realize that your stiff shoulder is not aggravated when you make a certain move. In the initial two phases, you must recognize that the joint is vulnerable; letting it heal, instead of forcing it to heal, is critical. Forcing the shoulder to move when it is not ready only makes it stiffer and more painful, which is why Tonya found her physiotherapy sessions so torturous. Understanding what phase you are in can help you to emotionally deal with the problem and to set realistic expectations around your healing.

A frozen shoulder must be treated gently. Anti-inflammatory medication sometimes helps in its initial stages, but strong narcotics usually don't. I've had some success with corticosteroid injections to the joint, which decrease the pain and allow the patient to begin to resolve the issue by following the recommendations below. Gently and progressively stressing the soft tissues allows them to adapt. Sleep is also essential, as it gives the body time to repair.

MANAGING A FROZEN SHOULDER

- Apply heat during the freezing phase. Hot water in the shower or a warm pack in your armpit works wonders. Acupuncture can also be very helpful.
- Let your arm hang with gravity and perform Shoulder Pendulums (page 109). Distracting the joint by using gravity to separate its bones can provide great pain relief.
- Go to your local pool, stand so your shoulders are submerged, and gently move your arm around in the water. Don't swim just yet. The buoyancy of the water allows you to activate the weakened shoulder muscles and will reduce pain.
- Do your Supine Shoulder Isometrics. (See the Shoulder and Arm Routine for Acute Pain on page 108.)
- If your frozen shoulder is really painful, try sleeping in a recliner chair for greater comfort, or put your affected arm inside your shirt so it can't get away from your body during sleep.
- Don't force range of motion. Allow it to return naturally.
- Remind yourself that 95 percent of the time, a frozen shoulder resolves. The pain is temporary.

One of the keys to dealing with a frozen shoulder is accepting that you have a vulnerable shoulder. Don't try to make your arm do something it can't. Giving your body a chance to heal while keeping the muscles activated is like sitting in an idling car at a traffic light. Keep it warm until the light turns green. Your frozen shoulder will resolve eventually, so be nice to yourself and your shoulder, during the freezing phase in particular. It will speed up the recovery process.

When your range of motion improves and you enter the thawing stage, you're ready to move from the Shoulder and Arm Routine for Acute Pain to the standard one (page 101). At first, adjust the range of motion exercises to stay within a pain-free range, or at most a pulling or stretching type of discomfort. Use the numeric pain rating system (NPRS) to monitor your progress. You should see the NPRS trend down over time, not up. If the NPRS is 3 or lower, you can continue the program, but if the NPRS is 4 or greater, it's good to scale back and refrain from pushing the activation and range of motion so aggressively. Decrease your active range of motion, and decrease the intensity of your contractions from 80 percent down to 40–50 percent until your NPRS is 3 or less.

Tennis Elbow and Golfer's Elbow: How the Shoulder Affects the Rest of the Arm

Two of the most common wear and tear conditions that affect the upper extremity are tennis elbow (pain on the outside of the elbow) and golfer's elbow (pain on the inside of the elbow). You do not have to be either a golfer or a tennis player to suffer from these tendon breakdowns. Any repetitive activity that involves your arms can put you at risk, particularly if you have forward head posture and a poorly positioned scapula. I looked after a very famous drummer with golfer's elbow, and he had no time to enjoy golf; he was far too busy beating his drums while on tour. Playing the drums is a very physical activity, and the years of performing had caught up with him. Fortunately, his tendon was not significantly damaged, and a combination of injection therapy, acupuncture, and restoring his Foundation for Movement helped him to keep performing his magic.

When there is a failure of the Foundation for Movement in the head, neck, and upper back area or in your shoulders and arms, there is a significant increase in force that occurs in the distal part of the arm—the part closest to the hand—in fact, up to three times the force! Whenever someone has wrist, hand, or elbow pain, I always—yes *always*—look up the kinetic chain at the shoulder and cervicothoracic spine. You can have the best therapy to treat your tennis elbow or wrist tendonitis, but if you do not restore your foundation in the shoulder, head, and neck, the problem is likely to remain.

Tennis and golfer's tendonitis are similar degenerative conditions of the forearm's tendons caused by repetitive motion; they just affect different tendons. They work like this: Repetitive motion—like hitting that drum a thousand times—causes your forearm muscles to tighten, weaken, and shorten. These shortened muscles then start to pull on the extensor carpi radialis brevis (ECRB) tendon, a wrist extensor, in the case of tennis elbow, or the flexor carpi radialis tendon, a wrist flexor, in the case of golfer's elbow. In both cases, collagen fibres start to tear. Picture the ECRB tendon, for example, as a rope being pulled in two directions, some of its strands fraying under the pressure. Tear enough of its collagen fibres and you'll reach a tipping point and a tear will emerge in the ECRB tendon itself.

In an effort to fix the tear, the body fills the area with inflammatory granulation tissue, a substance used to heal wounds. The granulation tissue creates that tenderness and pain you feel when you move your arm. The first step in recovery is to take the tension off the rope—the fascial chains that travel throughout our body. Releasing the tension from the shoulder, up the kinetic chain, goes a long way to restoring the regenerative cycle, allowing the tendon to heal. The vast majority of these injuries heal without surgery.

As with all bodily wear and tear problems, we need to ask why they've occurred in the first place. An abnormal shoulder position changes how we use our arm muscles. To avoid shoulder pain, we will change how we use the arm, which overloads the forearm muscles. Combine this with the additive effects of repetitive movement described above and we have a recipe for body breakdown. The affected part of the arm depends mostly on your activity: tennis elbow for the outside (lateral tendon), golfer's elbow for the inside (medial tendon). The solution is the same for both problems: Work all the way along the kinetic chain. Mobilize the thoracic spine, correct forward head posture, and then release the muscles that support the shoulder girdle. In some cases, you may have to go even further along the kinetic chain to the pelvis and hip to correct tennis or golfer's elbow, but that is rare. The beauty of this approach is that you can change part of your body that is not painful, and it will accelerate the healing of your elbow.

Our shoulder routine starts with an exercise to release the back of the shoulder, followed by a dissociation technique. It's important to lengthen the tissues around the shoulder, before activating them with dissociation techniques to break bad movement patterns. The following shoulder routine will stimulate remodelling of tissue around our shoulder, activate the important muscles, and teach them to work in the proper way, so that injuries heal and pain resolves. The shoulder in particular is vulnerable to poor activation sequences because there are so many players involved. There are approximately 17 muscles that attach to the scapula; they not only have to turn on, but they must work together and grow strong enough to protect our arms. The spine and the shoulder blade have to be stabilized and move in the correct fashion to set the rotator cuff up for good function. Don't worry, I have you covered: Just follow the exercises in the routine and you will hit the pain-free jackpot as your foundation returns.

Shoulder and Arm Routine

Pain in the shoulders, elbows, or wrists is a common occurrence in those who use their upper bodies a lot—whether working on a computer or cleaning the windows. The culprit is often related to certain muscles working less than they should, particularly the deep muscles found in the shoulder and forearm. This Shoulder and Arm Routine wakes up these neglected and hard-to-reach deep muscles to restore balance and keep you moving pain free.

The first time you perform any new exercise, focus primarily on following the technique cues provided. Don't worry so much about counting reps. Once you feel you have a basic grasp of the exercise, start your first set slow and gradually increase how hard you contract your muscles. Work toward increasing your range of motion for the exercise. Rest for 30 to 60 seconds between each set and between exercises.

IF YOU DON'T HAVE SHOULDER OR ARM PAIN: Cycle through the Shoulder and Arm Routine along with the other routines according to the Movement Longevity Schedule (page 196) that best accommodates your lifestyle.

IF YOU DO HAVE SHOULDER OR ARM PAIN: Perform the Shoulder and Arm Routine for Acute Pain and the Head, Neck, and Upper Back Routine for Acute Pain (page 87) if your NPRS is 7 or more. Perform the Shoulder and Arm Routine and Head, Neck, and Upper Back Routine (page 75) on alternating days for four weeks if your NPRS is 6 or less. You should notice a significant decrease or complete elimination of pain, at which point you should continue with the Movement Longevity Schedule (page 196).

Posterior Shoulder Active Self-Myofascial Release

Loosens the tissues at the back of the shoulder while activating many shoulder muscles for greater freedom of movement.

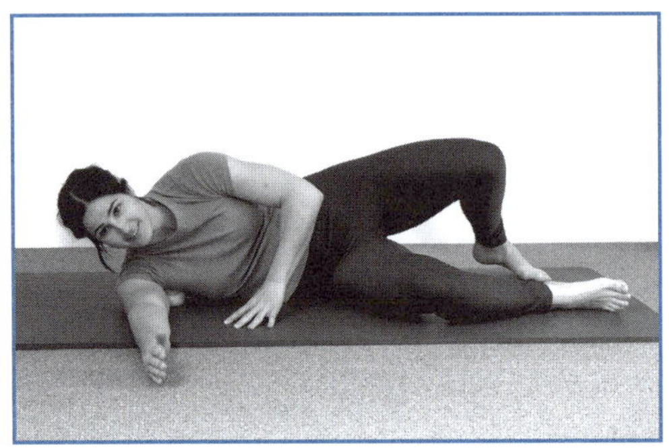

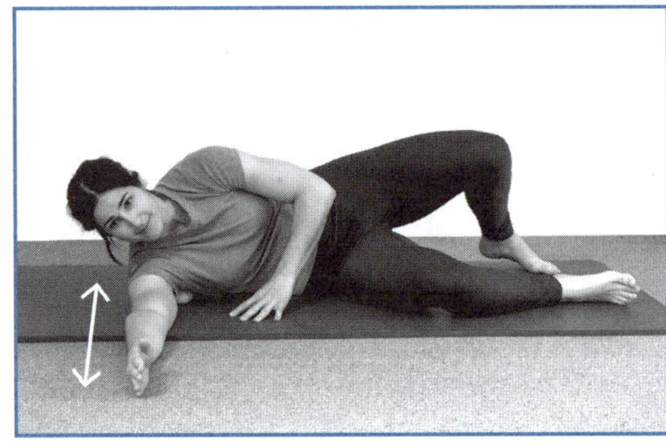

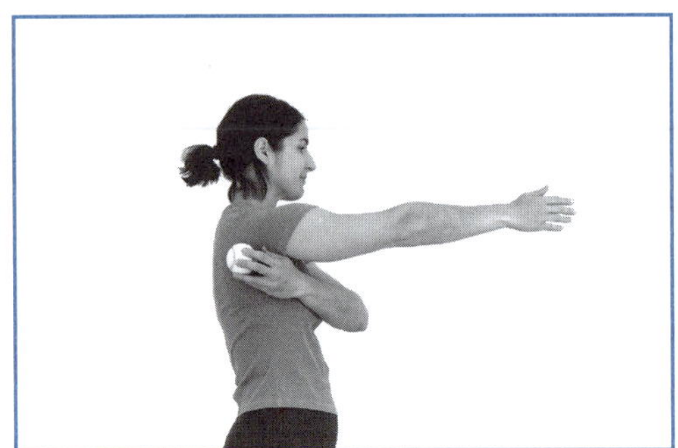

1. Lie on your right side with your right arm perpendicular to your body. Start all of these movements with your working arm perpendicular to your body. Place a massage ball under the meaty area just behind your right armpit. Do your best to keep your muscles relaxed while resting on the ball. You can control how much pressure you apply with how much of your body weight rests on the ball.

2. First, pretend your arm is a drawer: Moving your right arm from the shoulder, reach your arm away from your body (opening the drawer) and then pull it back (closing the drawer). Repeat three times.

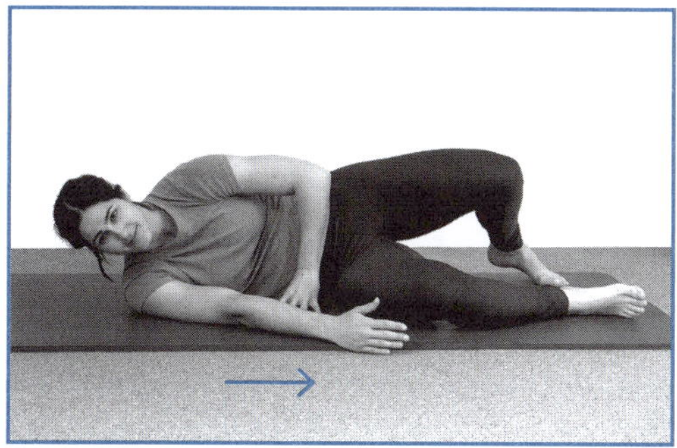

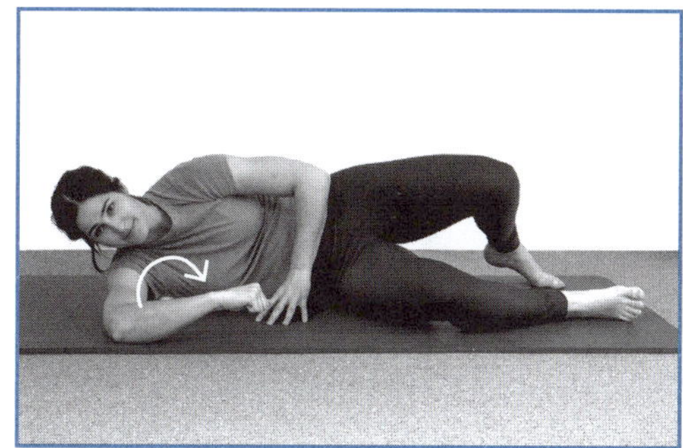

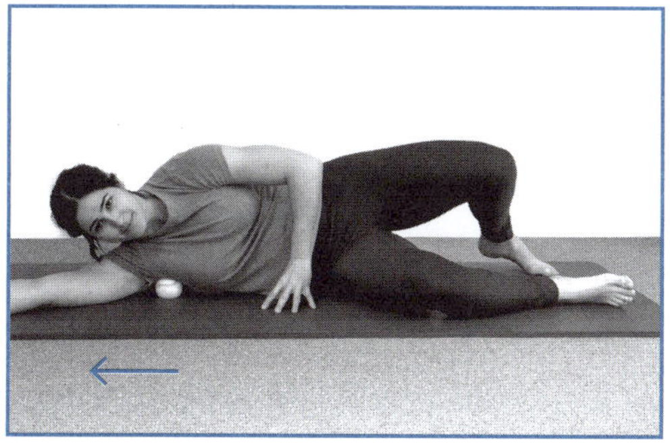

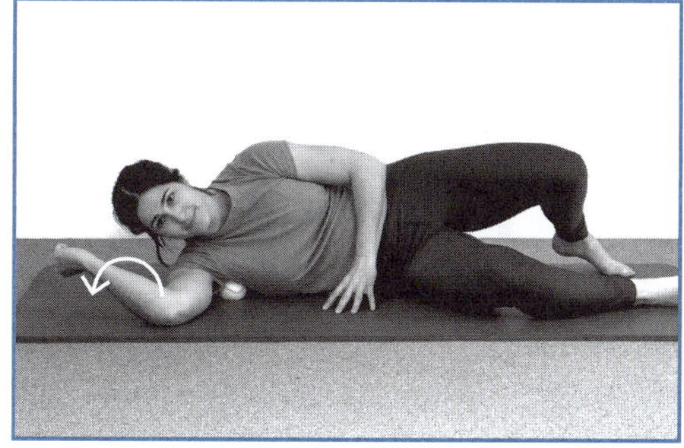

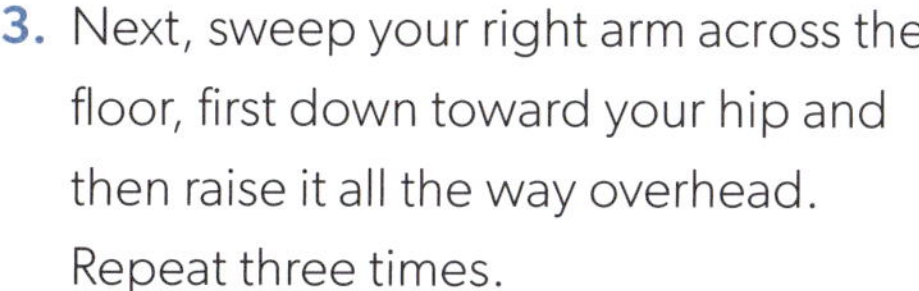

3. Next, sweep your right arm across the floor, first down toward your hip and then raise it all the way overhead. Repeat three times.

4. Next, rest your right elbow on the floor, bent at a 90-degree angle. Rotate your shoulder so your hand moves like a windshield wiper. Attempt to touch the floor with the back and then the front of your hand. Repeat three times.

5. Repeat steps 2 to 4 after moving the ball under an adjacent meaty area behind your armpit. Repeat again with the ball under a third meaty area behind your armpit.

6. Repeat steps 1 to 5 on the opposite side.

Slumpy Serratus Activator

Restores activation of a key stabilizer muscle of the shoulder that is often neglected and can be hard to contract with more conventional exercises. Also opens the chest and improves shoulder posture.

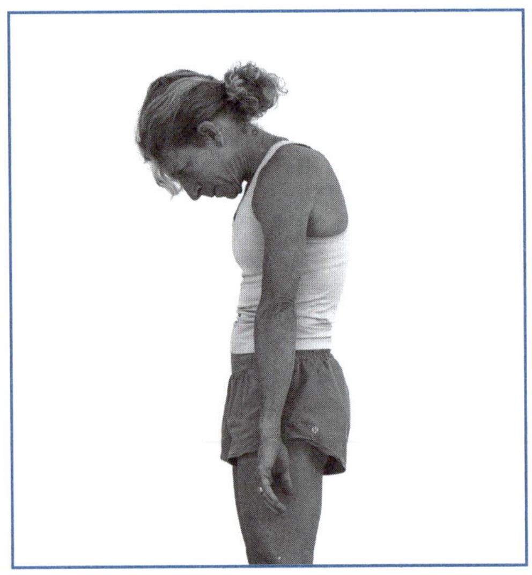

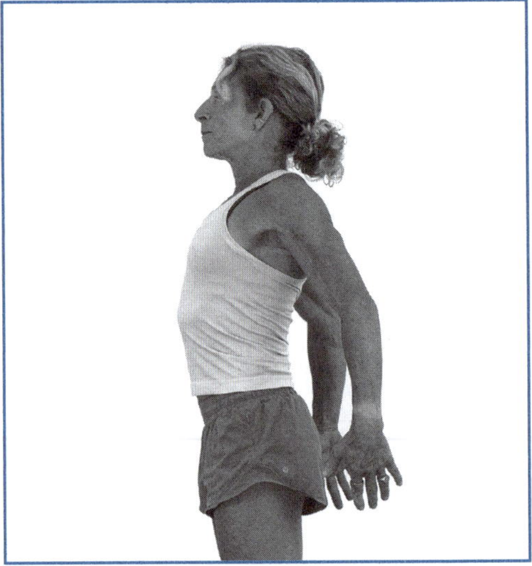

1. Stand in poor posture with your spine curved in a C shape and your chin toward your chest.
2. Move into good posture while reaching your arms up behind you, with your palms facing each other and your shoulder blades pulled together, in toward your rib cage. Keep your shoulders relaxed and away from your ears. Maintain a tall spine and continue to squeeze your shoulder blades together. Hold for 10 seconds.
3. Perform two sets of four reps each.

Scapula Circles

Mobilizes your shoulder blades through their full range of motion to unlock movement that is often lacking.

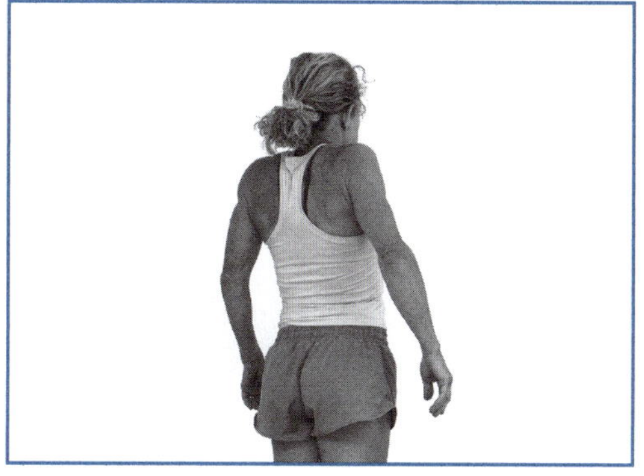

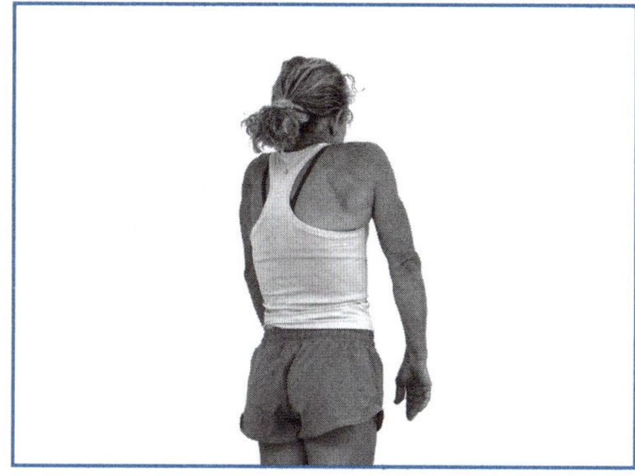

1. Allow your arms to dangle loose throughout the exercise. Lift your shoulder blades as high as possible.
2. Keeping them up, move them as far forward as possible.

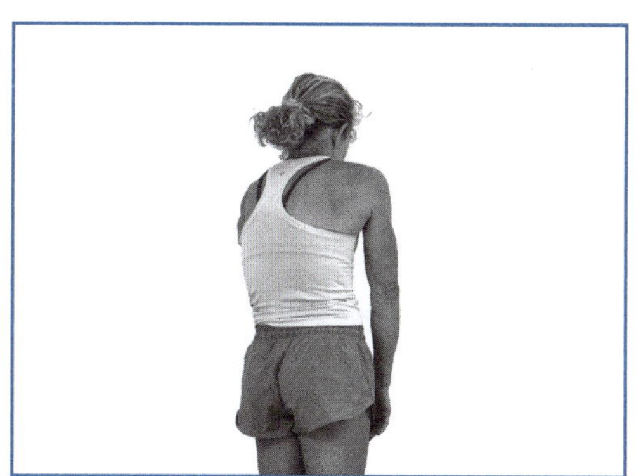

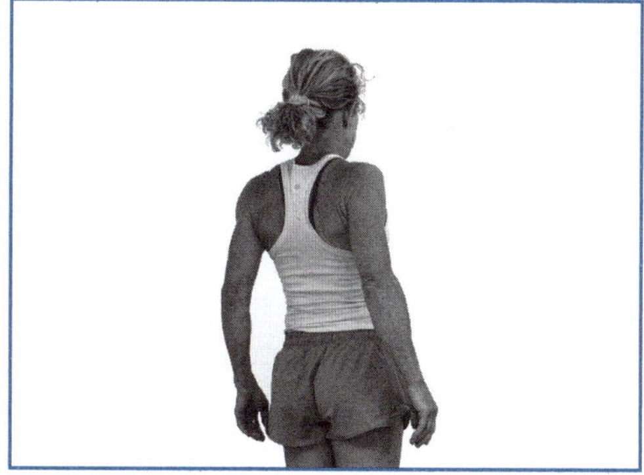

3. Keeping them forward, move them down as low as possible.
4. Keeping them down, pull them back as far as possible.
5. Keeping them back, lift them as high as possible.
6. Perform two sets of four reps each.

Extended Elbow Wrist Fan

Wakes up deep muscles of the forearm and elbow and restores stability to the entire kinetic chain from wrist to shoulder.

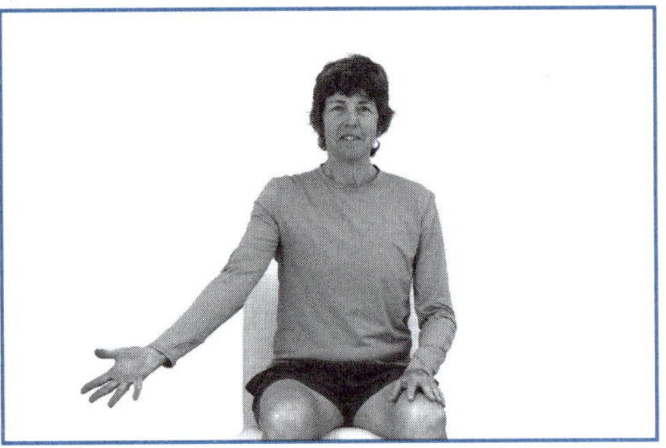

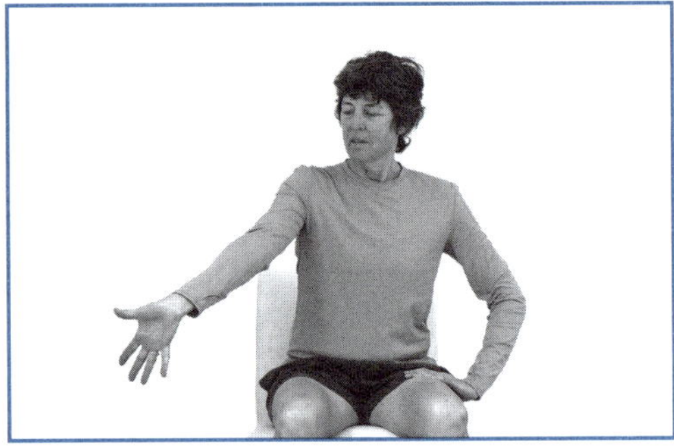

1. Start with one arm just in front of your body with your elbow in full extension and fingers straight and flared out wide.
2. Contract your biceps and triceps, and extend the wrist so your palm faces forward. Hold for five seconds.

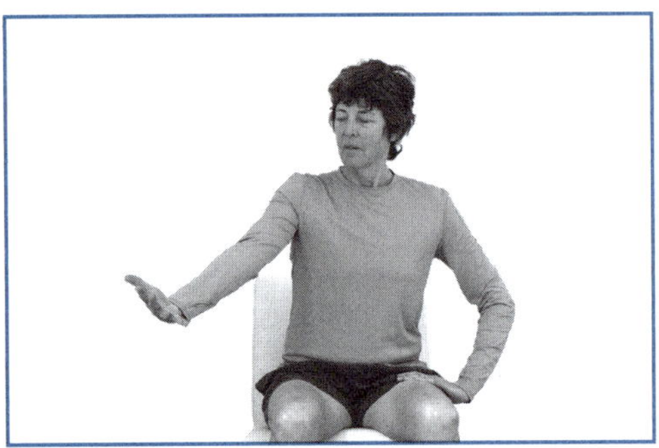

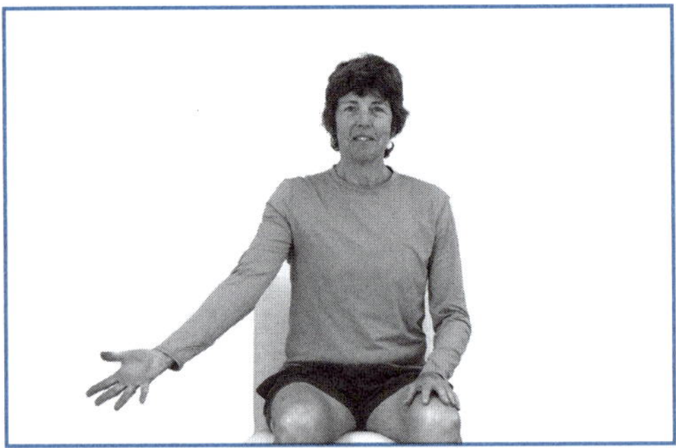

3. Keeping your fingers straight and flared, flex the wrist as much as possible so you can see your palm. Avoid cupping your palm; keep the hand flat. Hold for five seconds.
4. Return your wrist to a neutral position as you gradually relax all of your muscles.
5. Repeat eight times, holding each muscle contraction for five seconds.
6. Repeat the exercise on the opposite arm.

Shoulder and Lumbar Flexion Dissociation

Resets a common movement pattern where the low back compensates for a lack of shoulder mobility. Reduces the risk of low back pain and improves shoulder movement.

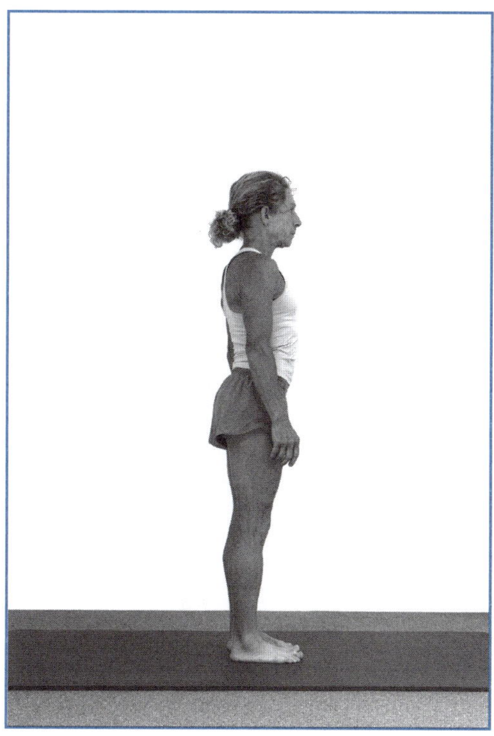

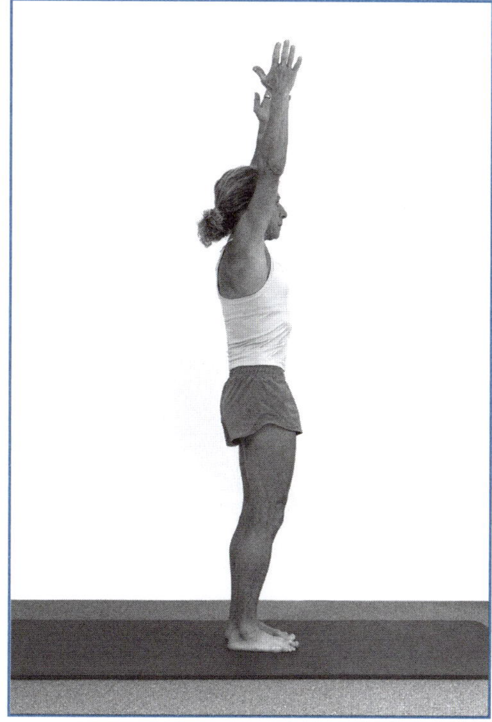

1. With your arms by your side, extend your low back and tilt your pelvis forward as if you had a tail and you were sticking it up in the air.
2. Lift your arms in front of you, bringing them all the way overhead, while simultaneously rounding your low back and tilting your pelvis as if you had a tail and you were trying to tuck it between your legs. Hold for five seconds.
3. Slowly return to your starting position.
4. Repeat steps 1 to 3 eight times.

Shoulder and Arm Routine for Acute Pain

If your NPRS rating is greater than or equal to 7, start here until your pain reduces and you feel comfortable to perform the standard Shoulder and Arm Routine (page 101). Complete this routine in the morning after you get up, at lunchtime, dinnertime, and again before bed.

Wrist Circles

Mobilizes the wrist through its full range of motion and gently wakes up the stabilizer muscles of the shoulder.

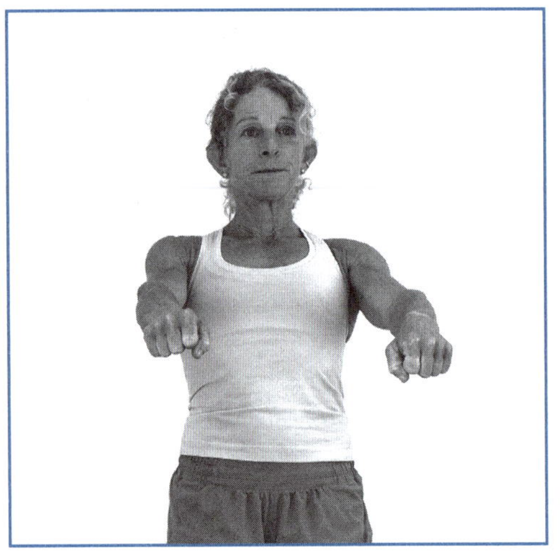

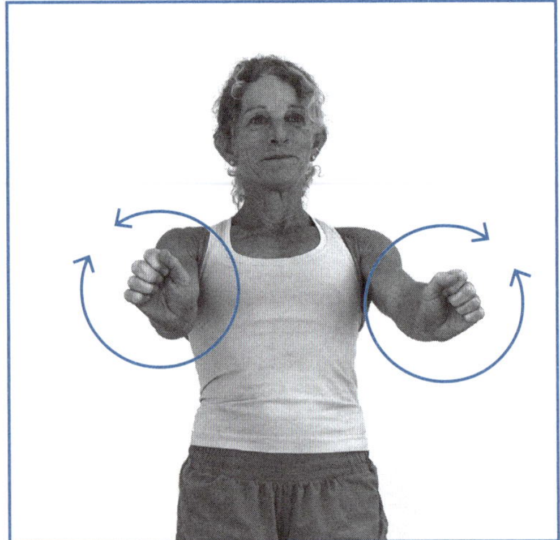

1. Gently make fists and extend your arms out in front of your body. If your shoulder is in so much pain that you cannot hold your arm in position, do the exercise with your arms at your sides.
2. Without moving your shoulders, slowly draw a circle with your fists, moving through as wide a range of motion as possible without exacerbating pain.
3. Perform five circles in each direction.

Shoulder Pendulums

Gently relieves tension in the shoulder muscles and decreases pain.

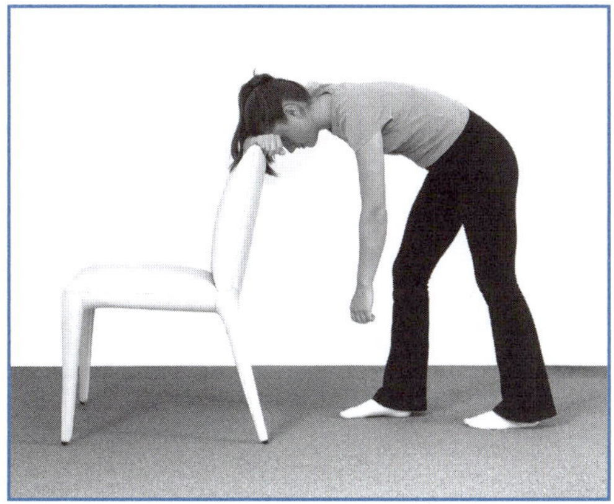

1. With the painful arm hanging loose, bend over and support your body weight with your opposite arm or your head resting on a chair, table, or other stable surface.

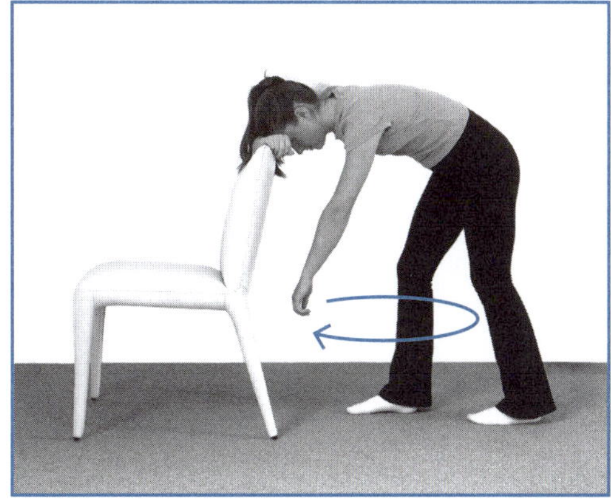

2. Slowly and gently move your painful arm in a clockwise circle five times while breathing in and out to facilitate muscle relaxation.

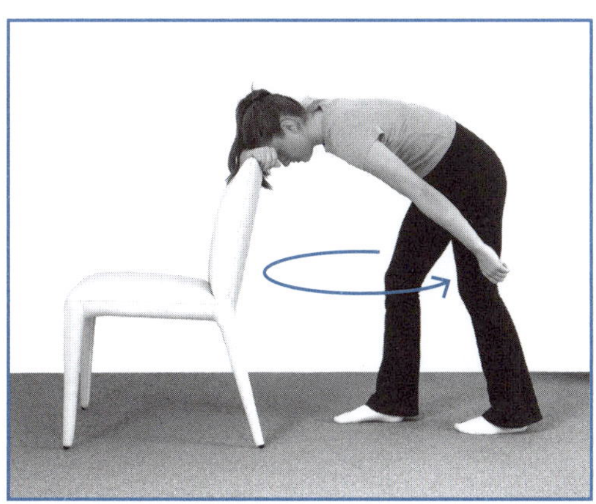

3. Pause, and then repeat moving counterclockwise.

Standing Shoulder Isometrics

Gently wakes up the muscles of the shoulder that can help alleviate acute shoulder pain and increase range of motion. Working both the painful and the pain-free arms provides a neurologic crossover effect that improves strength on your painful side by up to 40 percent.

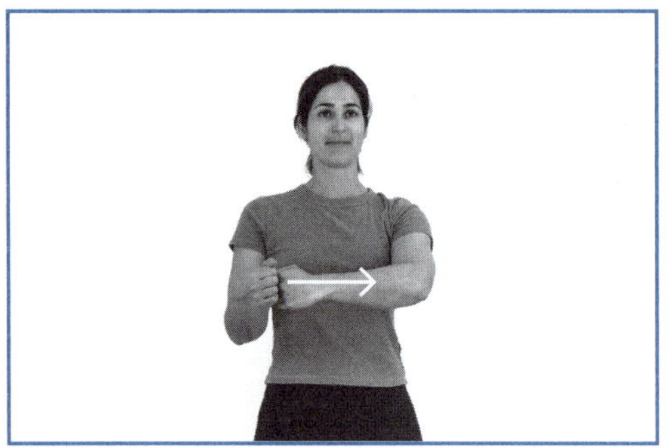

1. Stand tall and bend the elbow on the painful side to about 90 degrees in front of you. Gently make a fist. Place your opposite fist on the inside of your wrist, and use your painful side to press into the fist for five seconds.

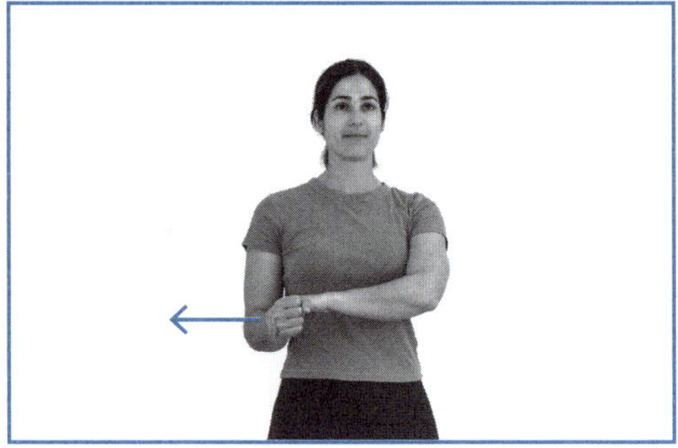

2. Grasp the wrist of the painful side to hold it in place. Use the painful side to press outward for five seconds.

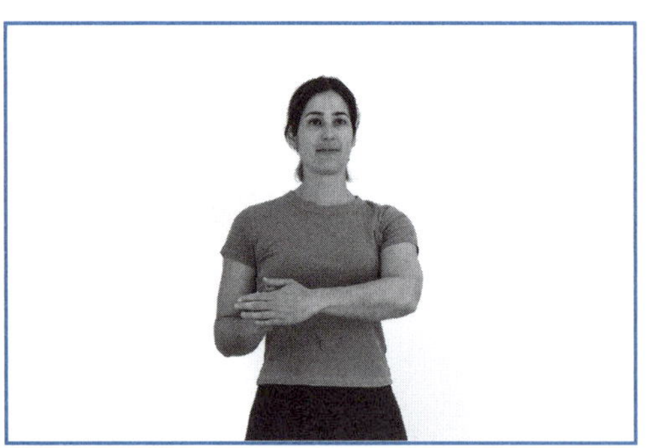

3. Place your palm on the top of your fist to hold it in place. Use the painful side to press forward for five seconds.

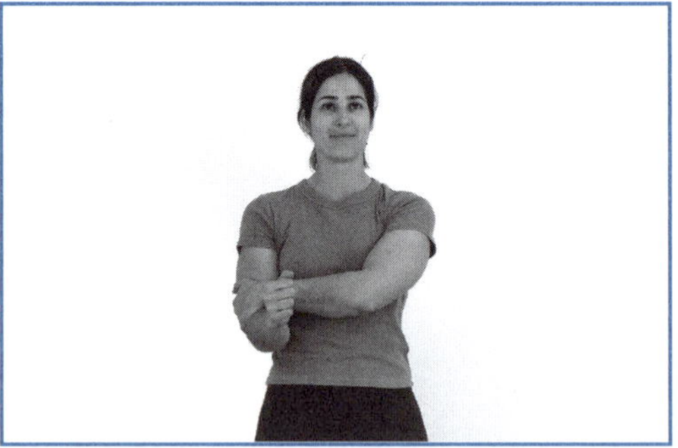

4. Wrap your opposite hand around the elbow on the injured side. Press your elbow into your hand for five seconds.
5. Repeat steps 2 to 4 four times.
6. Repeat on the pain-free side.

Counter Stretch End-Range Expansion

Safely and progressively increases your shoulder flexion range of motion and stability.

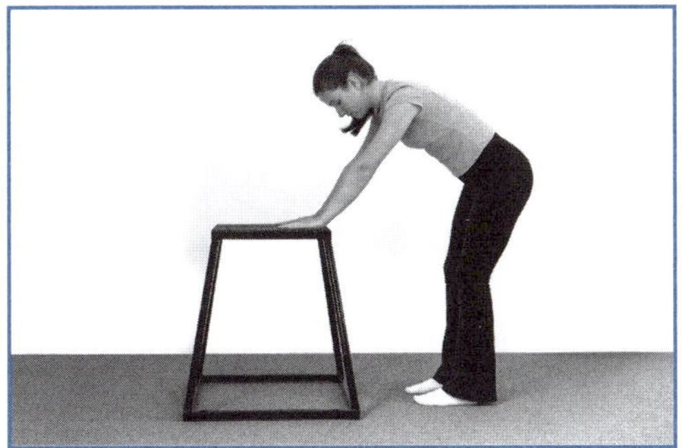

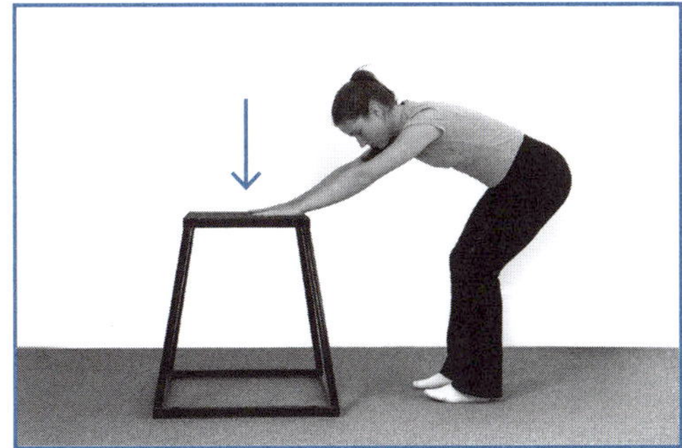

1. Stand an arm length away from a stable surface at about waist height (e.g., a tabletop or counter). With your feet shoulder width apart and your knees slightly bent, extend your arms and place your hands on the surface at a level that doesn't exacerbate your painful shoulder.
2. Gently bend your knees as you sink your buttock backward, as though you are taking a seat. While you are doing this, press the palms of your hands into the stable surface. Only go to a point of comfortable stretch in your shoulder; it should not be painful.

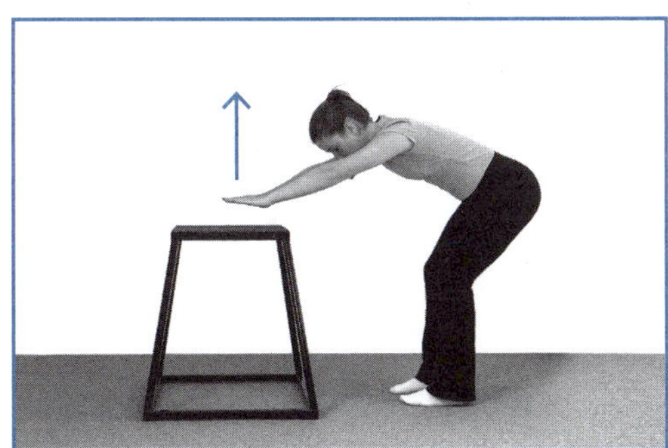

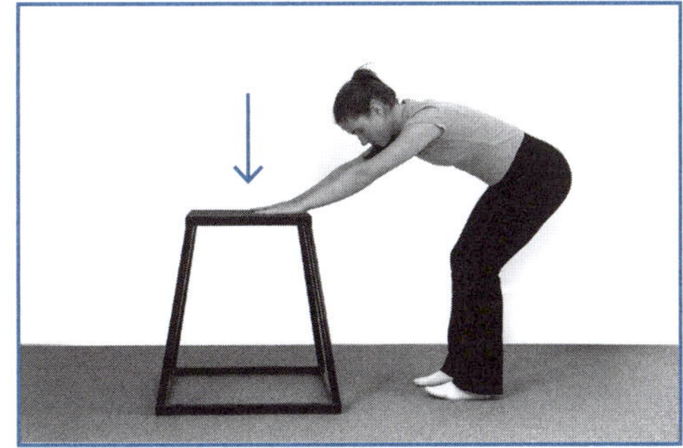

3. Lift both hands off the table as high as you can (it may be only a millimetre) and hold for five seconds. Try to lift the hand of the painful side a few millimetres higher each day.
4. Return your hands to the table. Press into the table for five seconds. Then return to the starting position.
5. Repeat four times.

CHAPTER 7

Lower Back and Hips

If you lack a foundation in your hips and lower back, you are not alone. Challenges in these two areas almost always go hand in hand because they play off one another. Wear and tear issues in the back and hips are extremely common, so I didn't get to feel special when I developed low back and buttock pain postpartum. I explained earlier about my abdominal hernia—how the tissues between my rectus abdominus muscles had stretched to accommodate my large babies, and how that extra tissue eventually remodelled when I practised using it properly. Still, I was left with a weak core, poor pelvic floor function, and stiff hips because my psoas muscles were on vacation.

The psoas is one of the muscles responsible for stabilizing your spine and pelvis when you are sitting and standing, so if it is not working well, you will not maintain proper alignment of your pelvis and hip joints. Oh, and glutes, what glutes? When I reflect back on my residency days when I only jogged for exercise, I know I developed the typical imbalances that long-distance runners get: poor gluteal muscle development, tight hamstrings, and posterior pelvic tilt. Throw on top of that postpartum core weakness and I was a ticking time bomb for back pain.

Forget about postpartum weakness for a moment. Sitting is probably the number one culprit for hip and spine pain. When we sit, the psoas muscle is shortened and becomes tight and weak. This sends signals to our glutes to shut down, leading to tight hamstrings, and that changes the alignment of the pelvis. We lose three pillars of our Foundation for Movement with poor tissue pliability, a change in joint alignment, and poor gluteal and psoas muscle activation. These changes affect the active range of motion of our hips and the small joints in our spine, too, which means all four pillars are affected.

Depending on your specific alignment, activities, and imbalances, you could wear out a disc, your hip, a facet (one of the small joints in your back), or simply have painful, tired muscles in your back and buttocks. If you are really unlucky, all four! Eighty percent of the general population will have at least one episode of significant back pain in their lives, and one in four people will develop hip osteoarthritis. So, let's look at the hip and pelvis relationship in a little more detail.

The alignment of the pelvis and the spine are very important for normal function. When the alignment is off, it's called pelvic tilt. Imagine you have a tail: A posterior pelvic tilt means that the tail would be tucked between your legs, while an anterior pelvic tilt is the opposite, with the tail touching your back. If the psoas isn't working correctly, you will notice an abnormal pelvic tilt. Imagine bringing your knee up toward your chest, like when you put on a pair of socks. You might automatically move into a posterior pelvic tilt because the tissues in your butt are too tight, pulling at your legs and restricting their motion. If the muscles that support the neutral alignment of the hip and pelvis are too weak, we lose stability and more movement occurs through our lower back instead of the hip. You may find that you stand with your "tail between your legs" in a posterior pelvic tilt or that you slump when you sit. We start to believe that these postures are taking pressure off our bodies, but actually these compensations can lead to wear and tear in both the hip and the spine, causing muscle pain, hip impingement, early arthritis, labral tears in the hip (tears in the ring of fibrocartilage that lines the hip joint socket), or abnormal stress on the discs and the small facet joints of the spine. Disc degeneration, herniations, and eventually arthritis of the spine or hip could be in your future.

During my pregnancies, I experienced pain in my lumbar spine and sacroiliac joint. (The SI joint is where the pelvis and spine meet.) My core was weak, and right after the kids were born, I was always carrying them around, which often led to an imbalance in how I stood, accentuating a posterior pelvic tilt and even a lateral tilt of the pelvis as one child was always sitting on my hip!

One day I made a wrong move, and my back went into spasm. I could not bend or sit. Muscle spasms in your back happen when the body is trying to protect you. All the muscles turn on so that they will splint the joints in your back. Knowing that doesn't make it any more pleasant when it happens, though. I felt pretty good after a few weeks of rest (to the extent possible with two kids under two years old), but I lacked mobility in my spine and hips. I got really sore and stiff and was not able to do much active movement for several weeks—until I began addressing the pillars lacking in my hips and core.

Just like with my sore neck, I went for massages and often felt better afterwards, temporarily. I knew that my core was weak, so I started doing exercises and quickly realized that I always felt better once the muscles were turned on and activated. I began experimenting on myself with different routines. The biggest challenge was figuring out how to improve the mobility of my spine while avoiding those terrible back spasms. I was a little fearful that if I made the wrong move, I would drop to the floor in pain. If you've experienced extreme back pain, you can probably relate to the feeling.

The key turned out to be releasing tight tissues and immediately following up with muscle activation to provide stability to the spine. One of the worst things you can do for your back is release all of the soft tissues without then activating the muscles to protect the spine. Having the mobility without muscular control is a recipe to freak out your nervous system. If you move into your new range of motion without using the correct muscles to stabilize the spine, the brain perceives danger and automatically turns on the muscles in your back—that means spasms. It's important to go slow and steady. First tackle the poor tissue pliability of the small muscles of the spine, followed by activation of the deep spine stabilizers.

Activating your muscles in an isometric fashion, holding good pelvis and spine alignment, is very safe. Once you begin to improve the mobility of the hips and small joints of the spine, it's time to address movement patterns. Releasing the tight hip capsule and muscles in my buttock and activating my psoas and glutes were critical steps in my recovery.

I always felt better after I did the exercises. At first, the benefits would only last a day, as I would subsequently do something to overload my spine again, but after about four to six weeks of doing the routines, my pain was essentially gone. I would get up in the morning and not feel so stiff. I had to do these routines, and I still do before I play sports, to maintain body balance. The effort of doing the exercises for 15 to 30 minutes per day is worth it for me to be able to participate in the things I love to do.

Even with this daily maintenance, the muscles in my left pelvis and spine still have a propensity to shut off. This is due to the way I move playing tennis, a sport that involves a lot of stopping and starting and changes in direction. How I sit doesn't help much either. Like most people, I slouch sometimes. At first, I found it disheartening when the issue would recur after I thought that I had fixed it. I would feel great for months, even years, and then my pain would come back. Unfortunately, it is not possible to prevent every ache and pain if we live an active life. Each one of us is a work-in-progress. Even if you have some bad habits or some wear and tear around a joint, you can keep yourself healthy and active by tending to your Foundation for Movement. We *can* change how we move and give our bodies what they need to keep us active and to reduce pain over the years.

DO YOU HAVE A TIGHT HIP POCKET AND/OR SPINE DEFICIENCIES?

1. Lie on the floor with your legs stretched out straight.
2. Use your hands to pull one of your knees up toward your chest. Observe if you can touch your knee to your chest without the opposite thigh coming off the floor.
3. Can you bring your hip up past a 90-degree angle? If you can flex your hip beyond 90 degrees, when doing so does your knee point to your armpit or to the outside of your shoulder?
4. Test the opposite leg.

If you cannot flex your hip beyond 90 degrees, the resting leg comes up off the floor, or your knee points to the outside of your shoulder, do the Low Back and Hip Routine (page 124).

DO YOU HAVE A WEAK CORE OR LOW ENDURANCE?

1. Lie on one side with your shoulders, hips, and legs in a straight line. Stagger your feet, so your top foot is in front of the bottom and both lie on the floor.
2. Position your forearm closest to the ground perpendicular to your shoulder.
3. Lift yourself off the ground with your forearm into a side plank and hold for 30 seconds.
4. Test the opposite side.

If you cannot hold yourself off the ground for 30 seconds, follow the Low Back and Hip Routine (page 124) to improve your core strength.

Never Too Late

Eighty-eight-year-old Dolores was the family matriarch. She had raised four boys, had eight grandchildren, and had been married to her childhood sweetheart for more than 60 years. She and her husband were pig farmers, the salt of the earth, and Dolores was deeply involved in the farm's day-to-day work: tending the vegetable gardens, preparing meals, and minding the pigs.

Dolores's back pain began with the birth of her first baby. With each successive child, the pain got worse. After the birth of her fourth, she was laid up for a month. Still, Dolores kept working, which meant a lot of bending and lifting. The pain would usually settle after a few days of rest, but those were few and far between on the busy farm.

After years of physiotherapy and back pain that got worse and worse, Dolores learned she had arthritis, but with all her nerves working, she wasn't a candidate for surgery. From there, things deteriorated. Dolores was incapacitated by pain. Even day-to-day tasks like cooking left her reeling, and she was taking more and more morphine. By the time her son came to me, her family was beside themselves. Dolores was in such excruciating pain that she was bound to a wheelchair and so stoned on narcotics that she could hardly speak. She had a big problem, complicated by drugs, inactivity, and poor fitness.

For many, drugs play an integral role in pain control. But for Dolores, the morphine was detrimental. Not only did it do nothing for her pain, it also made it impossible for her to do anything for herself. I helped wean her off them, eventually swapping the powerful narcotic for regular Tylenol. Once Dolores regained her faculties, she began the movement foundation program—relaxing and rebalancing the muscles in her hips and back with massage and acupuncture, and then reprogramming her muscle-firing patterns.

After years of pain, however, Dolores had a psychological struggle too. She had to learn to differentiate between the good pain and the bad and keep the former from impeding her progress. She had to recognize what her fear of pain had cost her and consider the emotional toll of losing her independence. The healing process was hard—and sometimes painful—but it was necessary for her to regain her health.

Each day, her family took her for short walks and got her into a pool to walk and float. While floating, the small muscles in the spine don't have to fight gravity, which allows them to relax and the pain to dissipate. Dolores knew that the severe arthritis in her spine would remain, but how she viewed and approached her pain could change.

As she gained understanding, she gained confidence. Learning how to work with her pain, her fears and doubts eased. She learned how to move slowly and steadily, what activities to do and which ones to avoid. She was growing stronger and more independent each week, her pain becoming less and less. It was wonderful to watch her change.

Dolores is an amazing example of true grit. And a reminder to us all that despite a lifetime of intermittent back pain, it is possible to persevere and work with our body to have a relatively pain-free and happy life. Even if you fall off the wagon, you can get back on. Don't stop moving; just change how you move! One year after we first met, Dolores brought me a gift from her garden: bright red roses.

Going Deeper

Lori is 59 years old and trained as a social worker. She sits all day while working with her clients. Many years ago, she was really active in ballet, but she has become more sedentary. She has suffered from occasional mild low back pain over the years but nothing that prevented her from working or doing any activities.

Lori got up in the middle of the night to get a glass of water, and a series of unfortunate events transpired. She didn't see her dog and almost stepped on him. This caused her to lose her balance slightly—just as she was sneezing. A twist, a slight forward bend, and the increase in abdominal pressure as she sneezed created the perfect combination for an acute spinal-disc herniation.

Lori could barely move. She got into bed with a searing hot pain radiating down the back of her left leg from her buttocks to her toes. She could wiggle her toes and bend and straighten her knee, but anything that put a stretch on her sciatic nerve, like a straight leg raise, sent her through the roof. She had numbness in her left foot and had to limp because of the pain and weakness that she felt in the leg.

The spinal disc is a specialized structure that sits between two bony vertebrae and acts as a shock absorber. It has a unique structure: A tough outer layer, referred to as the annulus fibrosus, surrounds a soft gelatinous central area known as the nucleus pulposus. The disc structure is analogous to a car tire: Strong, thick rubber surrounds the flexible inner tube that contains the air. You can imagine drilling a hole in the thick outer rubber, causing the inner tube to spill out. This is exactly what happens with a disc herniation. The annulus is made of tough collagen fibres that can break down over one's lifetime, particularly if you have a weak core and weak hip muscles. This leads to abnormal wear on the annulus, and progressively some of the fibres tear. As the annulus tears, the nucleus pulposus material herniates into the defect.

You may have heard this referred to as a "slipped disc." There are different grades of tearing with a progression: An initial bulging of the central nucleus material into the defect is known as a disc bulge; a protrusion is when the disc material pushes out against the annulus, which then begins to extend into the spinal canal, applying pressure on the spinal cord or nerve roots. If there is a complete tear in the annulus, the disc material herniates into the spinal canal and applies pressure on the local nerve roots—a disc herniation. The final stage is sequestration, which occurs when the disc material completely extrudes out of the disc and sits freely within the spinal canal.

With each stage of disc pathology, there is an increased risk of damage to the local nerve root. Leg pain is caused by pressure exerted by the herniated disc material on the sciatic nerve. The pressure may only cause pain, but if the pressure is excessive, particularly in very large acute herniations, there can be loss of nerve function.

Imagine that the nerve is a highway. A car rolls down the nerve highway carrying information that is dropped off at the end of the line. The car heads back the way it came carrying a different load, more information telling the nervous system what to do. Applying pressure to a nerve is like blocking the road so traffic can't get through. When the instruction to contract doesn't reach the muscle, it is paralyzed. With an acute herniation, sudden pressure is applied to the nerve, and it doesn't have a chance to adapt. In Lori's case, the herniation was abrupt.

Disc disease developing over time creates a different scenario. When it occurs over years and decades, there is a very slow and progressive increase in pressure on the nerve roots. This slow-going gives the cells in the nerve a chance to adapt to the increased pressure, so the information is able to get down the leg to the muscle, with no paralysis. In essence, the body builds a side road to bypass the area of compression or blockage, allowing information to flow freely, however abnormally, to the lower leg.

Lori had paralysis of the tibialis anterior muscle, the muscle that pulls your foot up toward your torso. She felt pain when I lifted her leg straight up by the heel, which indicated that there was irritation and excess tension on the sciatic nerve. Her reflexes were normal. An MRI confirmed she had a disc herniation at L4/L5, with a large sequestered disc fragment sitting within the spinal canal and applying pressure to the L5 nerve root.

Management options included rest, heat, gentle range of motion, a nerve block and/or epidural cortisone injection, or surgery. Oh, and of course, exercise. It generally takes six weeks for the acute pain to resolve and several months for the nerve function to regenerate. Some surgeons advocate for the removal of the large disc fragment when there is a sequestered disc and motor loss. There is evidence that surgery will speed up the recovery time, but ten years down the road, the results are identical with regard to function and persistent low back pain whether you have surgery or not. During the long wait time for surgery, the herniated disc can atrophy and no longer cause symptoms. The time it takes for the piece of disc material to dissolve depends on how large it is and where it is.

Regardless of whether or not you have surgery to remove a disc fragment, it is imperative that you change how you load your lumbar spine. You need to change the movement dysfunction that created the excess wear and tear on the spinal disc, so that your condition does not progress. When there is a loss of disc height associated with the damaged cushion, the alignment of the small joints (facets) at the back of the spine changes. With increasing stress on the small joints, arthritis can develop. As well, an increased load on the disc above and below the area of the initial herniation can lead to a progression of the problem along the spine. The best treatment is to unload the spine by improving the mobility and strength of the core muscles.

Lori did not have surgery, and her nerve function recovered over approximately nine months. She has occasional back pain if she doesn't do her exercises, but she is doing really well and has returned to some of her sporting activities.

From Back to Hip and Back Again

When your core is weak and your psoas is taking a break, it is very common to experience pain in either the back or one or both hips. Often times, one gets better, and the other flares. I find that people who do a lot of activities that involve twisting, changes of direction, and sudden stops and starts often have more pathology that settles in the hips. If we combine these types of movement with a little aging and sitting at a desk all day, it's a recipe for more hip than spine pathology.

Nick had limited mobility of his hips, and he lacked rotation, particularly internal rotation. What I have observed over the years is that often the tissues on the buttock right by the hip pocket are *way, way* too tight. The hip is a ball and socket joint. When we flex the hip by bringing our knee up toward our chest, the ball (or femoral head) has to sink back into the socket, or pocket if you will. If the connective tissues at the back of the hip are not supple enough, like the leather on a new baseball glove, then the femoral head will stay too far in front and pinch the tissues, causing pain as you flex your hip up. The hip pocket is kind of like the pocket in a baseball glove. A new glove's leather can be a bit stiff, and so the pocket for the ball is not as big, and it is harder to catch the ball and keep it in the glove. Once the glove softens, deepening the pocket, the ball sits very nicely in the glove when you make your catch. If you don't have a good hip pocket and you repetitively pinch the tissues, eventually you will tear something. The key is to centre the femoral head in the socket by creating a good hip pocket, so that it will stop pinching tissue at the front. Improving the tissue quality at the back of the hip to make space for the femoral head prevents abnormal loading of the joint. Persistent abnormal loading can lead to hip impingement (thigh and pelvis bones pinching), labral tears, and premature arthritis.

The exercise routine below will help to create a hip pocket and stop impingement, labral tears, and the arthritis train. The routine involves performing some ASMR to release that hip pocket and then activating key muscles to support your hip and back in making lasting changes in tissue quality.

Diving Down the Kinetic Chain: How Our Pelvis and Spine Affect Our Knees

Because we are connected from head to toe, it's important to consider how the joints adjacent to your spine and hips may be affected by a weakened Foundation for Movement. Knee pain is common, especially pain at the front (anterior) of the knee, and it can be difficult to treat. There are so many diagnoses to "explain" pain affecting the front of the knee; you may have heard reference to chondromalacia (softening of cartilage under the kneecap), subluxation and/or maltracking of the patella (the kneecap does not stay centred in its groove), knee tendonitis (jumper's knee), fat pad impingement (we all have a little fat at the front of our knee around the patellar tendon), or bursitis over the patella. We tend to focus on the knee and neglect *why* the knee is becoming painful, a point that I will emphasize in the next chapter, but often our knee is the victim of our hip and our foot and ankle.

So how does a problem with our hips lead to pain at the front of our knees? Here's an example of what I often see in my clinic. Meet Hannah, a 20-year-old college tennis player, who was keen to improve her game. The combination of drills, sprints, and heavy lifting overloaded the muscles in her right leg, and she developed pain at the front of her knee. This anterior knee pain was the exact condition she'd had during a growth spurt as a young teen.

Anterior knee pain is incredibly common, and one of the hardest pains to treat. Like most people's, Hannah's pain worsened after long bouts of sitting or going up and down stairs. Her knee wasn't swollen, nor did it lock, but it did catch sometimes. Only rarely did her knee feel like it would give way. She had a normal range of motion, but her vastus medialis oblique (VMO) muscle was underdeveloped—that is the muscle on the inside of the joint.

Most physicians would have told Hannah to rest until the pain resolved. If you follow that advice, you will feel better after a while, but your pain will return as soon as you get back to your activities. For Hannah, the problem was that the kneecap was overloaded, so we had to figure out why. Fortunately, there was no significant evidence of arthritis, and in the worst case scenario, she may have had some softening of the cartilage under the kneecap. Hannah didn't have a hip or back problem, but her case highlights the opportunity she had to avoid developing arthritis in her knees when she is 50 or 60 years old.

Luckily, I was acquainted with the four usual root causes of anterior knee pain: weak abdominal muscles, poor psoas function, lack of hip mobility (decreased internal rotation and tight IT band), and weak quadriceps muscle (particularly the VMO).

The psoas? You might be wondering why a muscle that flexes the hip and stabilizes the core might cause anterior knee pain. When the psoas is not working to stabilize our pelvis, the rectus femoris muscle (part of the quad) has to do double duty. The rectus femoris is known as the "kicking muscle," as it is responsible for extending the knee forcefully, but it also crosses the hip joint and can act as a hip flexor. When the psoas is not doing its job of stabilizing the hip and pelvis, the rectus femoris has to compensate. When it compensates, it becomes too tight and changes how the kneecap glides—or, in this case, doesn't glide—and voila: patellar overload and anterior knee pain.

The IT band, a dense piece of fascia that runs along the outside of the hip, is prone to tightness in anyone who does a lot of stopping, starting, and changing direction. An overly tight IT band changes the way the kneecap tracks, causing pain and wear and tear in the patellar tendon.

Every time Hannah played or performed drills, she was working her hamstrings and quadriceps *hard*. I was unsurprised to find both really tight, especially after learning that she rarely stretched or used a foam roller. Just like a tight IT band, tight hamstrings and quadriceps change the alignment of the knee, creating excess pressure and causing pain and wear and tear.

The final culprit was the underdeveloped VMO. With knee pain like Hannah's, the VMO often deactivates in response and starts to atrophy within 24 hours. A weak VMO can't absorb much mechanical stress, so the knee has to pick up the slack, enduring even more mechanical stress and worsening the pain that caused the VMO to shut off in the first place.

But wait—why was the IT band so tight? Looking at the joints above and below, I discovered that Hannah had very poor function of the muscles in her hip, glutes, and psoas, as well as very poor dorsiflexion of the ankle—a principle we will expand upon in the next section. So, the problem wasn't just the front of her knee; it had to do with how she used the muscles in her legs in general, her kinetic chain. Her movement pattern had overloaded her kneecap.

The Solution to Bad Hips, Low Back, and Even Knees

It can be frightening to try to move a stiff spine, particularly if you have splinted your back and moved as a block to protect it for decades. I get it. It is super helpful to get the hips moving better as improved mobility in the hips takes the stress off the spine and vice versa. Go slowly and gently. Like we saw with Dolores, some parts of your spine may not mobilize as well as others because there is too much deterioration and the changes have become fixed. That doesn't mean you can't make improvements. Just be sure you don't force the motion. Always listen to your back. If it does not feel right, then ease up. Start with the smallest of mobilizations and gradually ramp up the intensity of your muscle activations.

When you do a muscle activation, proceed in a progressive fashion: start with gentle contractions at about 20 percent activation, and gradually increase over time to your maximum contraction. Monitor your symptoms and how you feel. Our spines are made to move, so getting all of the muscles engaged and being sure that the multiple ligaments, joint capsules, and discs are pliable make the best recipe for a healthy spine. If you are not moving through one part of your spine, the levels above and below will wear out as they are exposed to increased stress. So, if you have a segment that is too far gone, protect the segments above and below by establishing your Foundation for Movement. Gently working through the exercise program that follows. Using your muscles to support your spine will go a long way.

Treatment to help loosen the tissues around your spine and pelvis can be helpful. If you go for a massage, be sure to activate your deep core muscles right after the massage so you can control the range of motion that your spine gained after the tissues relaxed.

Lower Back and Hip Routine

Many conventional approaches focus on the symptoms of pain and muscular tightness, but with this Low Back and Hip Routine, you'll get to the root causes, including a lack of mobility and deep muscle function in the spine itself as well as surrounding joints, to reduce and prevent pain.

The first time you perform any new exercise, focus primarily on following the technique cues provided. Don't worry so much about counting reps. Once you feel you have a basic grasp of the exercise, start your first set slow and gradually increase how hard you contract your muscles. Work toward increasing your range of motion for the exercise. Rest for 30 to 60 seconds between each set and between exercises.

IF YOU DON'T HAVE LOW BACK OR HIP PAIN: Cycle through the Low Back and Hip Routine along with the other routines according to the Movement Longevity Schedule (page 196) that best accommodates your lifestyle.

IF YOU DO HAVE LOW BACK OR HIP PAIN: If your pain is a 6 or lower on the NPRS, perform the Low Back and Hip Routine daily for two to four weeks. Once you notice a significant decrease or complete elimination of pain, continue with a Movement Longevity Schedule (page 196). If your pain is a 7 or higher on the NPRS, perform the Low Back and Hip Routine for Acute Pain two to three times daily until the pain decreases to below 7, and then follow the guidelines above.

Lower Back Active Self-Myofascial Release

Relaxes the muscles that often tense up and get sore in low-back-pain sufferers.

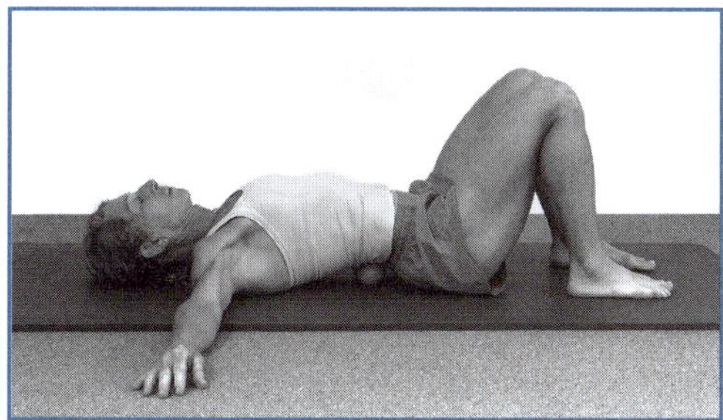

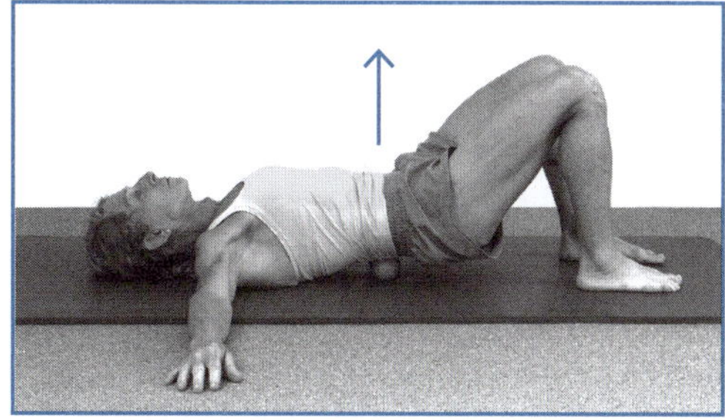

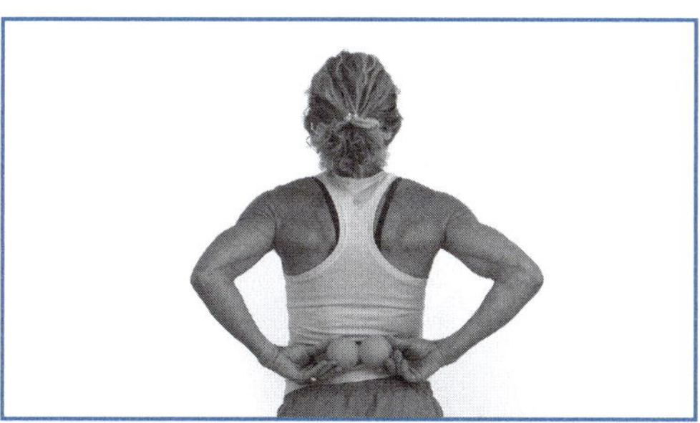

1. Lie down with your feet flat on the floor, and place a peanut ball or foam roller under your lower back just above your pelvis. If you use a peanut ball, it should rest on the muscles on either side of your spine. If you feel sensitivity in your back in this position, decrease the amount of pressure you are applying to the ball or roller by pressing through your feet, or adjust the position of the ball or roller so it is slightly above or below the sore area. Over about a week of doing this exercise, you will be able to move back toward the more sensitive area.
2. Tilt your pelvis up and down three times while maintaining contact with the peanut ball or roller.
3. Move your body so the peanut ball or roller is about one inch farther up your spine, and again tilt your pelvis up and down three times while maintaining contact with the peanut ball or roller.
4. Move the peanut ball or roller up another inch, and again tilt your pelvis up and down three times while maintaining contact with the peanut ball or roller.

Gluteal Active Self-Myofascial Release

Relieves tension in the gluteal muscles and helps release a tight posterior hip joint.

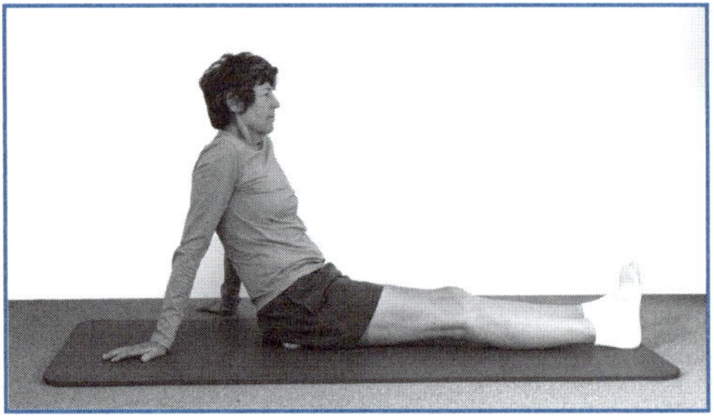

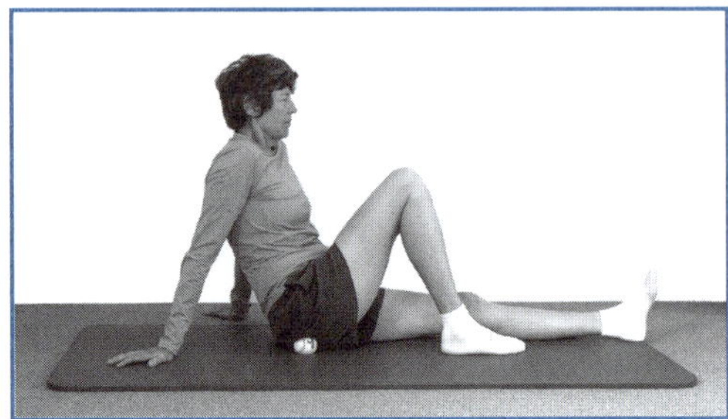

1. Sit with your legs extended out in front of you. Place a massage ball, golf ball, or any ball with a similar size and firmness underneath your right buttock.
2. Bend your right knee to place your foot flat on the ground. Your right knee should be pointed straight up.

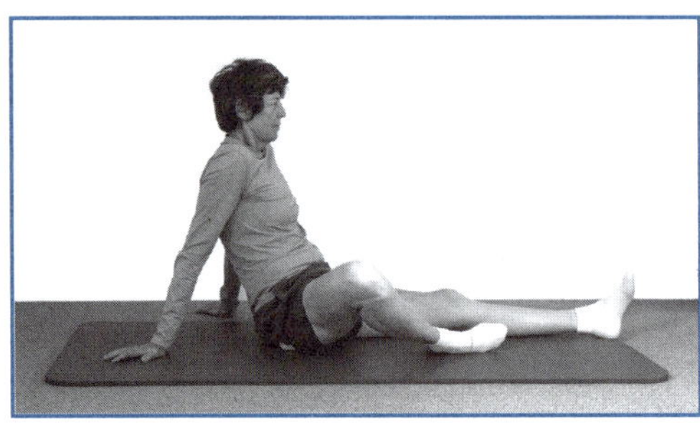

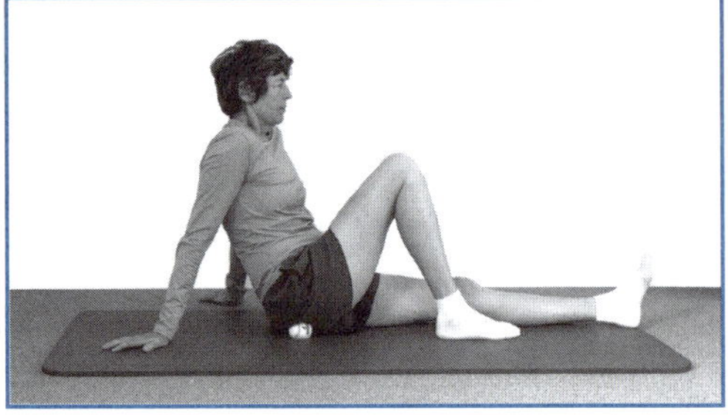

3. Slowly open your right hip to lower your knee toward the ground, and then bring it back to its starting position, with the knee pointed straight up. Repeat three times.
4. Keeping the ball in the same position under your right buttock, straighten your right leg out with toes pointed toward the ceiling, and then bring it back to its starting position with your knee pointed straight up and your foot flat on the floor. Repeat three times.
5. Move the ball to a different area of your buttock, and repeat steps 2 to 4.
6. Repeat steps 1 to 5 on your left side.

Birddog

Keeps the deep core stabilizer muscles active and strong. A must-do exercise for everyone, especially those who have had low back pain.

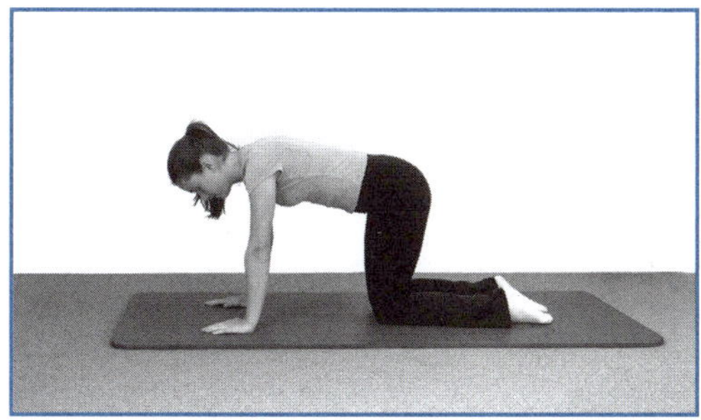

1. Start on your hands and knees with your hands directly under your shoulders and your knees directly under your hips. Your spine should be in a neutral position with your head facing straight down to the floor.

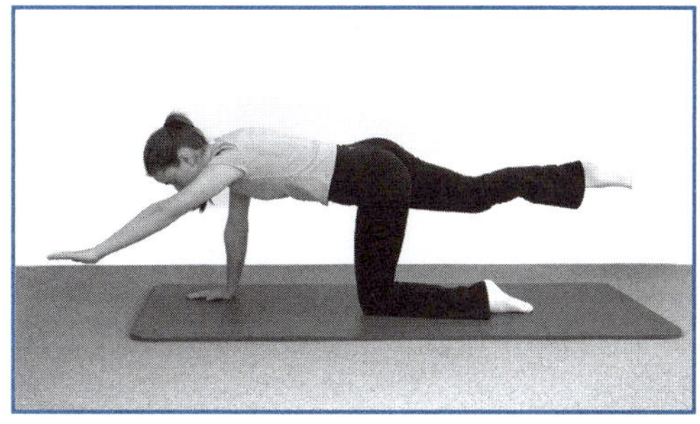

2. Slowly lift one leg off the floor until it is straight and more or less parallel with the floor. Lift your opposite arm up at a slight angle away from your head until it is also parallel with the floor. Hold for ten seconds, breathing naturally and keeping your core engaged and your body centred. Your torso should not shift up and down or side to side.

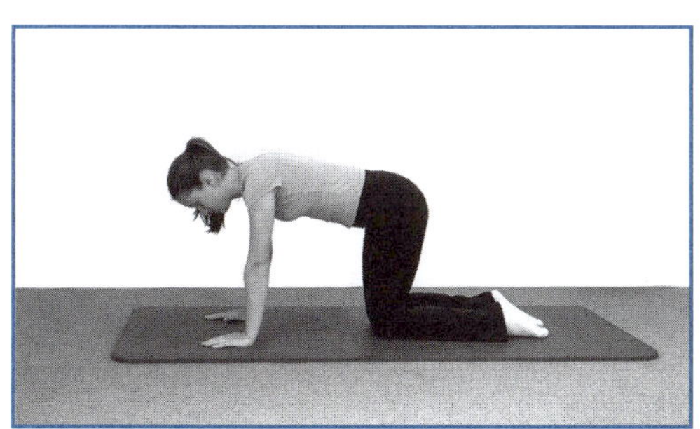

3. Slowly lower your arm and leg to the ground. Repeat six times.

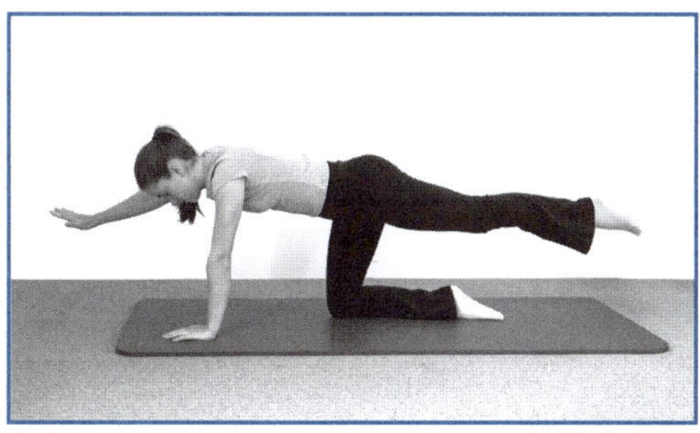

4. Repeat steps 1 to 2 with the opposite arm and leg.

Side Plank

Keeps the deep core stabilizer muscles working for a healthy low back.

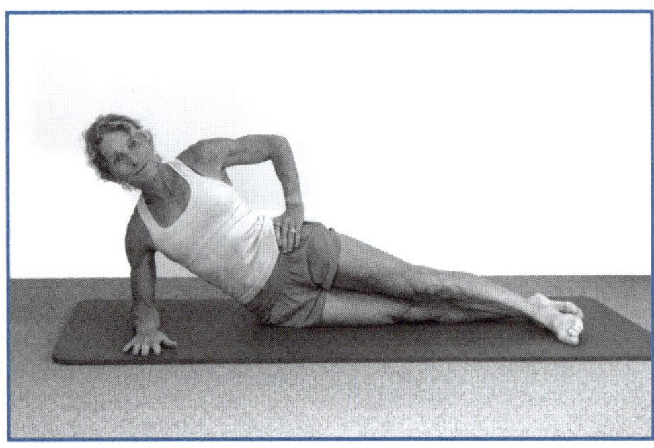

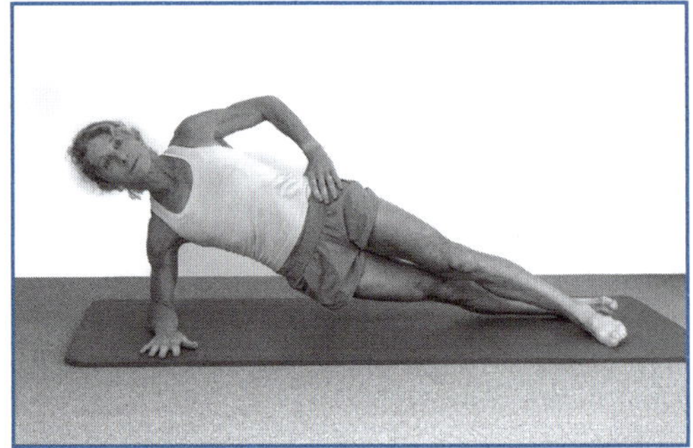

1. Lie on your side with your body straight and your elbow directly under your shoulder and your forearm on the ground, pointing away from your body. Place your top foot ahead of your bottom foot on the floor and allow the sides of your feet to rest on the ground. If this is too difficult to start off with, stack your legs with your knees bent at 90 degrees, and perform the steps that follow by pressing your knee into the ground instead of feet.
2. Pressing into your forearm and your feet, lift your hips up off the ground until your body forms a straight line. Hold for ten seconds while keeping your shoulders aligned with your body and relaxed. Breathe naturally. Lower slowly. Repeat eight times.
3. Repeat steps 1 to 2 on the other side.

Slumpy Psoas Activator

Wakes up a neglected muscle that plays a big role in keeping your low back, hips, and knees healthy.

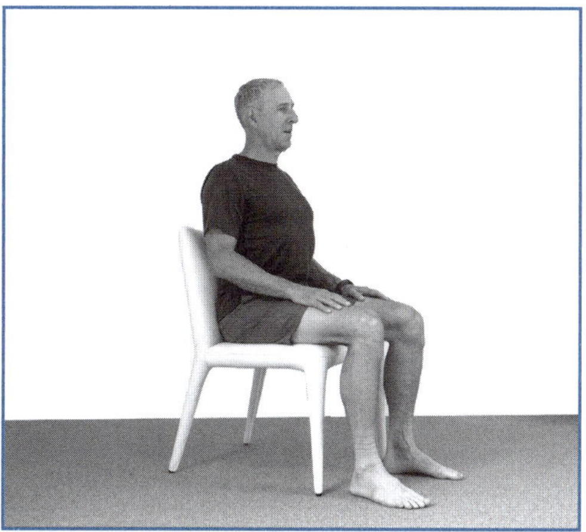

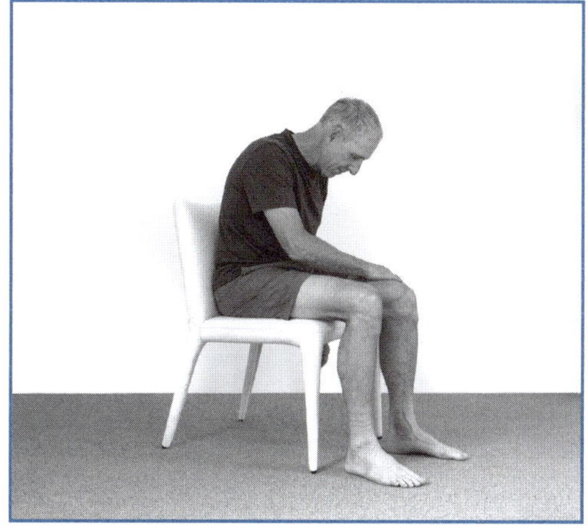

1. Sit on a solid chair or bench with your feet flat on the floor.

2. Position yourself with poor posture: curl your back into a C shape and allow your shoulders to slump forward. Lift one foot an inch off the ground. Place your opposite hand on the knee of the raised foot, and push your knee into your hand.

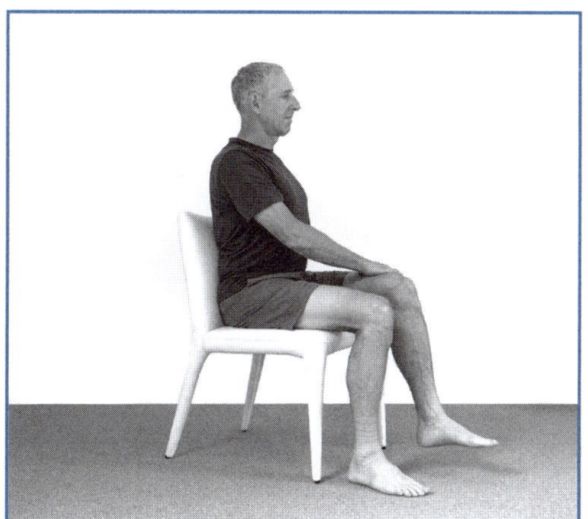

3. Keep your knee in position as you slowly sit up straight and pull your shoulders back into good posture. Maintain the pressure between your hand and knee for another five seconds. Slowly lower your foot to the ground. Repeat eight times.

4. Repeat steps 1 to 3 on the other side.

Neutral Hip Axial Rotations

The muscles that internally and externally rotate the hip are crucial for maintaining hip alignment and protect not only the hips, but our spine and knees. This exercise will get them turned on and tuned up.

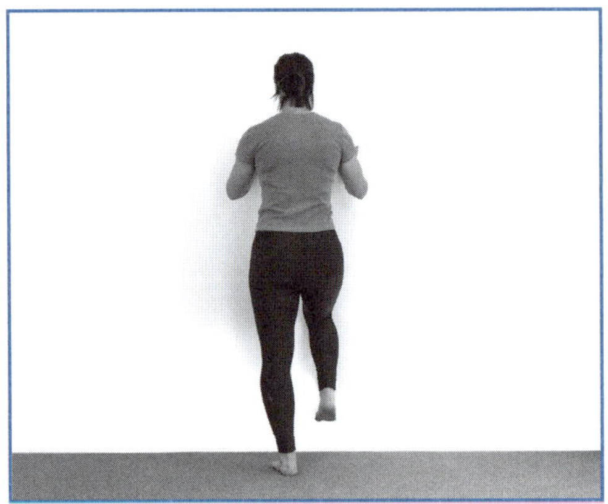

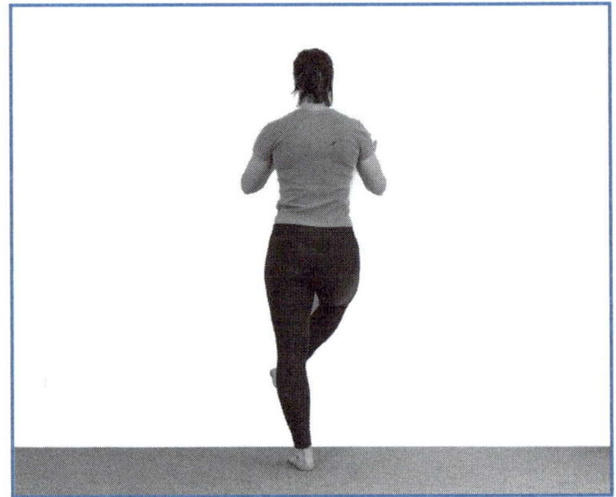

1. Stand facing a wall, just far enough away so that you can comfortably lift your hip and place your knee gently on the wall with your hip bent at about a 70-degree angle. Place your hands on the wall with elbows bent for support.
2. Moving from the hip, rotate the leg that is touching the wall so your foot points toward your midline. Hold for five seconds.

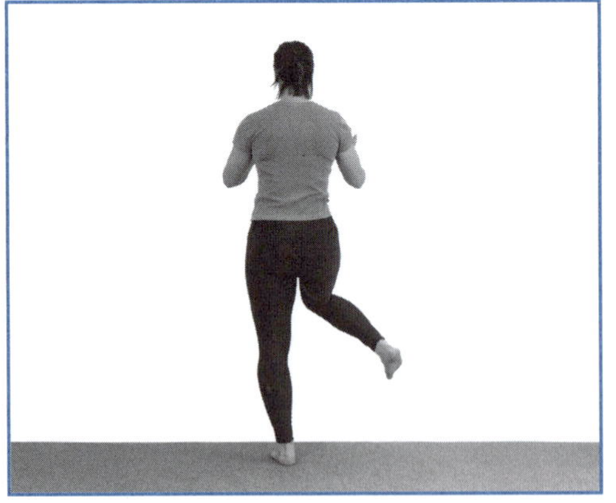

3. Rotate the same hip so your foot points away from the midline, and hold for five seconds. Repeat two times.
4. Place the knee two to three inches higher on the wall, and repeat step 2.
5. Repeat steps 1 to 3 on the other side.

Standing Glute Contraction

Our glutes are key muscles that so often fall asleep, particularly when we sit on them all day. Ideally you can take a break from your desk and stand up to do these contractions, but there is nothing wrong with firing up your glutes while you sit.

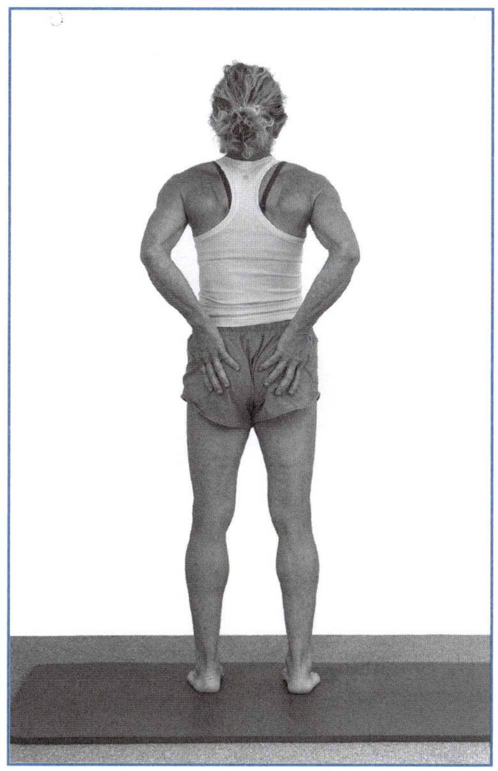

1. Stand or sit in good posture with your chin tucked, shoulders back, and feet shoulder width apart and pointing straight ahead.
2. Contract your pelvic floor muscles by pretending to stop peeing midstream. Pull your pelvic area up and inward.
3. Keeping your pelvic floor muscles engaged, contract your glute muscles and rotate your knees ever so slightly inward, gradually increasing the intensity of the gluteal contraction as much as you can without irritating anything. Hold for ten seconds, keeping your weight evenly distributed on your feet, both heel to toe and side to side. Gradually decrease the intensity of the contraction, and then relax completely.
4. Repeat six times.

Low Back and Hip Routine for Acute Pain

If you have back or hip pain greater or equal to a 7 on the NPRS, start here with the Low Back and Hip Routine for Acute Pain.

360-Degree Breathing

Gets your diaphragm working and relaxes hip and core muscles that often tense up with pain.

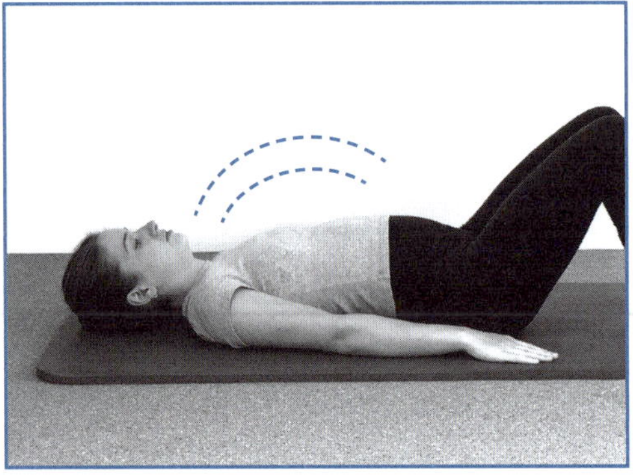

1. Lie on your back and relax your body.
2. Keeping your neck and shoulder muscles as relaxed as possible, close your mouth and inhale deeply through your nose. Imagine there is a balloon inside your chest, and imagine the balloon is expanding in all directions (360 degrees).
3. Slowly exhale through your nose, letting the air gradually release from your chest. Don't push the air out.
4. Continue this breathing technique for one minute.

Anterior Hip Active Self-Myofascial Release

Relaxes and brings kinesthetic awareness to the muscles in the front of your hip.

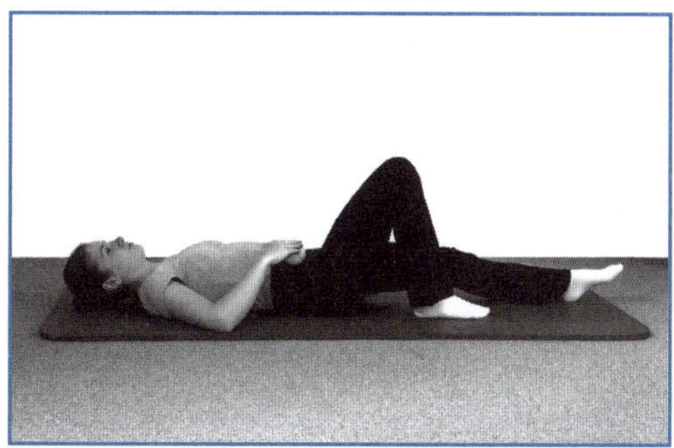

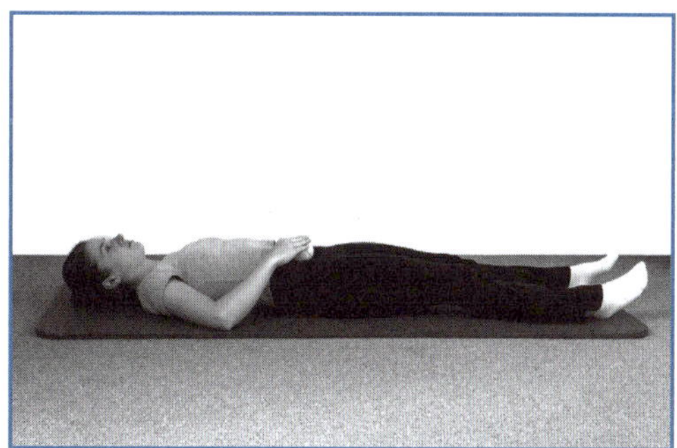

1. Lie on your back with one knee bent, and place a massage ball or weight (up to ten pounds) on the front of the bent leg's hip.
2. Apply pressure to the ball or weight with your hands, and then slowly straighten your leg.
3. Release some pressure from the ball, and return to the bent-knee starting position.
4. Move the ball to a slightly different area. Repeat steps 2 to 3 for one minute.
5. Repeat steps 1 to 4 on the other side.

Supine 90-Degree Hip Isometrics

Wakes up deep hip muscles that often go to sleep in response to pain.

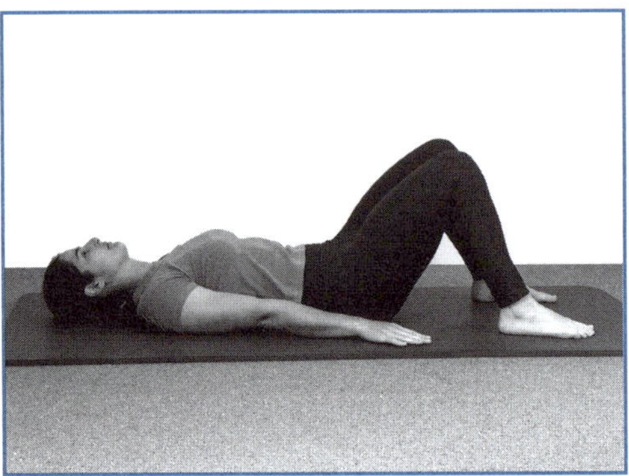

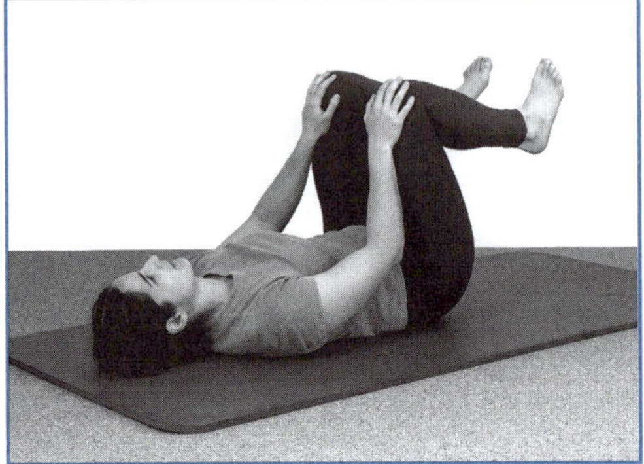

1. Lie on your back with your feet flat on the floor. Moderately contract your pelvic floor muscles by pretending to stop peeing midstream. Pull up and inward. Maintain this contraction for the duration of the exercise.
2. Lift up your legs so your thighs are at a 90-degree angle to your torso. Your lumbar spine should be in contact with the floor; you can gently press it into the floor during this exercise. Maintain this position for the duration of the exercise.
3. Place your hands on the front of your knees. Resisting the movement by maintaining your hip position, pull your knees toward your head. Hold for five seconds.

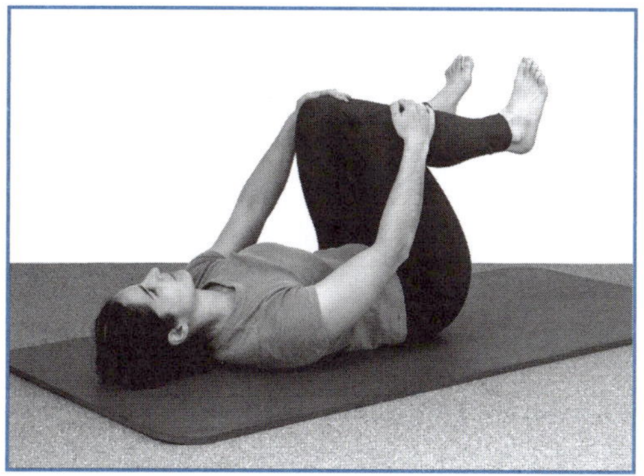

4. Hook your hands over the top of your knees. Resisting the movement by maintaining your hip position, push your knees toward your feet. Hold for five seconds.

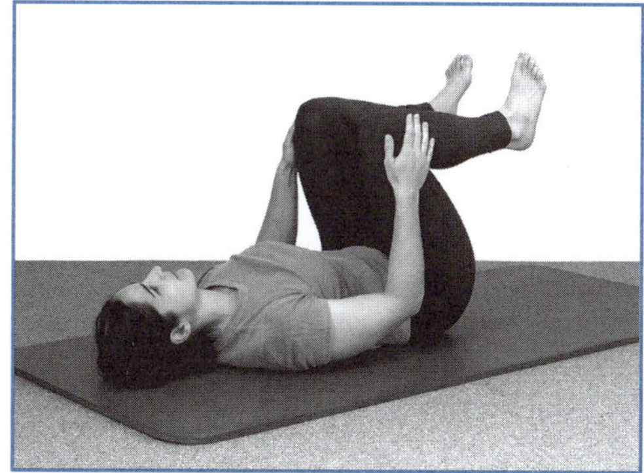

5. Place your hands on the outsides of your knees. Resisting the movement by maintaining your hip position, press inward for five seconds.

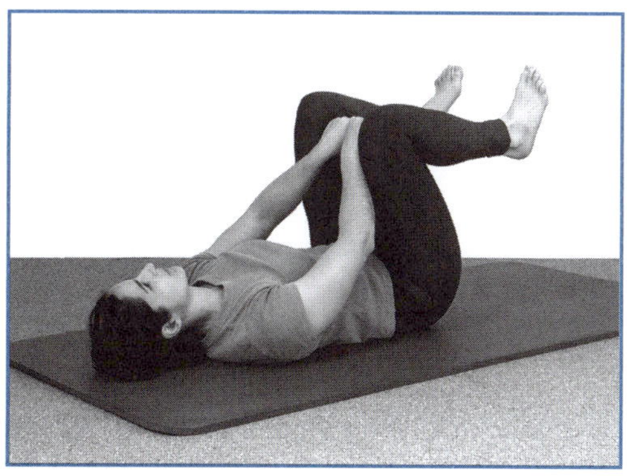

6. Make fists and place them between your knees. Resisting the movement by maintaining your hip position, push your fists outward for five seconds.

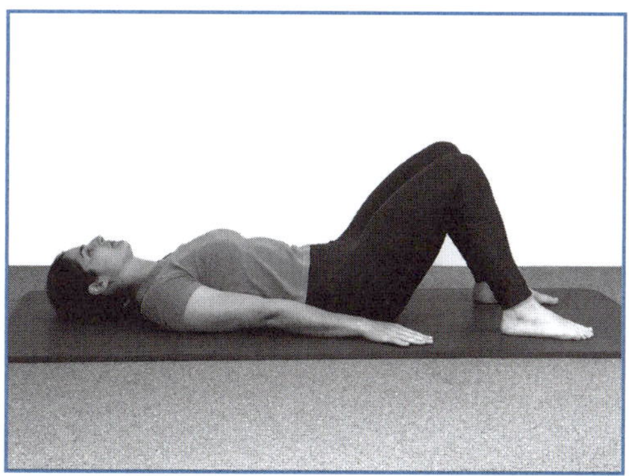

7. Lower your feet to the floor and relax.

8. Repeat steps 1 to 7 three times.

Abdominal Bracing

Activates all of the core muscles to provide stability to the low back and pelvis.

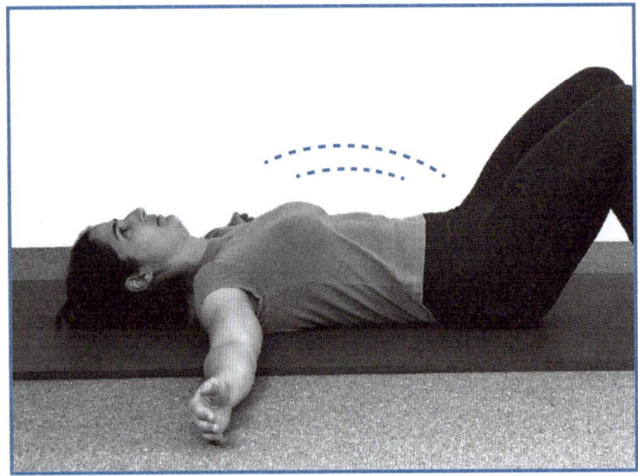

1. Lie on your back with your legs extended and arms relaxed by your side. Your knees and toes should be pointing toward the ceiling.
2. Contract your pelvic floor muscles by pretending to stop peeing midstream. Pull up and inward. Maintain this contraction throughout.
3. Imagine someone is about to punch you in the stomach, and contract your abdominal muscles to brace for the impact. Hold for five seconds. Relax.
4. Repeat steps 2 to 3 five times.

CHAPTER 8

Knees

The knee is the one of the most commonly injured parts of our body. It is the victim of movement dysfunction both above and below, meaning if you have problems with tight or weak hips or ankles, your knees will suffer. My first experience with knee pain was when I was a teenager. The pain was insidious. I noticed a little pain at the front of my knees when going up and particularly down stairs. Looking back, my knee pain was related to a couple of ankle sprains from playing basketball and the fact that I grew six inches in one year.

Back then, I played every sport I could. I loved basketball, volleyball, track and field, skiing, and tennis. And like most kids, I just wanted to play. No one told me how important a Foundation for Movement was or how to prepare my body for sports. We just hopped on our bikes and rode or jumped on the tennis court and played. The only thing going in my favour was that I did lots of different sports, so the varied movements helped keep my body in balance.

The growth spurt that I went through was great for basketball, but for a few months, I was a bit spastic, not accustomed to the new length of my limbs. I lost flexibility and did not gain strength at the same rate my limbs grew. Combine that with landing on someone's foot on the way down from a rebound, and I had a doozie of a left ankle sprain, with knee tendonitis (irritation of the tendon at the front of the knee) quickly following. Because of the ankle sprain, I'd lost ankle mobility, specifically dorsiflexion (closing the angle at the front of the foot and the shin), which automatically put more stress on the front of my knee. It was a perfect storm: My growth spurt led me to lose some of the Foundation for Movement I had built.

I did not formally test myself at the time (I didn't know any foundation tests back then), but I have had the chance to examine thousands of young active kids and learned that growth spurts make people vulnerable to injury. When you grow quickly, there is generally a loss of tissue pliability because the muscles, tendons, and fascia cannot keep up with the new length of the bones. I am not sure if you had flood pants when you were a kid, but I sure did. I grew like a weed, and it seemed like overnight the hem of my jeans was halfway between my knees and ankles. I thought my mom had put my jeans in the dryer and shrunk them. Imagine the tension in those jeans if they had been attached to my ankles as I grew. That is exactly what happens to fascia. Children need more recovery time after activity because they're still growing, and it's important to cycle through the foundational movement programs prescribed in this book to stay healthy. But growth spurts are only one factor; knee injuries can happen to adults too.

After the ankle sprain, I experienced a loss of flexibility in my muscles, combined with a loss of ankle dorsiflexion. I was placed in a cast for six weeks. My ankle got really stiff, and I never quite recovered the same degree of ankle motion I had before—until I started doing the Ankle and Foot Routine in this book (page 163). Remember that when we lose mobility at one joint, the joints above and below take on the extra load. If the ankle or hip is hurt, the knee has to work harder. The combination of less ankle mobility, poor flexibility, and, in retrospect, weak hips together doomed my knees for a dose of tendonitis.

The part of your knee that gets damaged will depend upon the shape of your bones and tendons; how you use your muscles; whether you lack mobility at the hip, ankle, or both; and how aggressively you move. Problems with the patellofemoral joint (under the kneecap) are extremely common, affecting over half of people experiencing knee pain in their teens. Others suffer from meniscus tears (which are shock absorbers in the joint; we have two in each knee), ligament tears (such as of the ACL), or damage to the joint surface (degenerative arthritis). Initially, the fix is the same for all of these knee conditions: restore mobility and strength to the hips and ankles and everything in between.

As a result of weak and tight hips and ankles, our quadriceps muscles often become too tight. The quadriceps consists of four parts, the deep intermedius along the centre of the thigh, the vastus medialis (VMO) on the inside of the knee, the vastus lateralis on the outside of the thigh, and the most superficial part, the rectus femoris. Not only are the quadriceps too tight, they are often really sore because all four parts do not work well together; often times the rectus femoris does most of the work. People become quadriceps dominant, which means they are also failing to use their gluteal muscles properly, resulting in tight, tired quadriceps. From there, imbalances around the knee often result in pain. If we ignore the root causes of our pain, we could develop further wear and tear in the joint that may eventually become arthritis.

DO YOU HAVE TIGHT QUADRICEPS AND HIP MUSCLES?

1. Find a firm surface where you can safely lie back and hug both knees to your chest with your buttock positioned just at the surface's edge. This could be your bed, the top of a staircase, a sturdy dining room table, or the stretching table at your local gym. With your buttock at the edge of the surface, release one leg at a time and let gravity pull it toward the ground. If your hip extends so that your leg is parallel to the surface, your psoas is not tight. If your knee does not naturally hang at a 90-degree angle and remains somewhat extended, your quads are tight. Finally, if your leg pops off to the side, the muscle at the side of your hip, the iliotibial (IT) band, is tight.

2. To determine if you are not using your gluteal muscles properly and are quadriceps dominant, take a picture of yourself from the side while standing naturally. Draw a line straight up from your ankle (centred on the outside ankle bone or fibula). Your hip, shoulder, and ear should line up perfectly with one another. If your hips sit in front of the line, you are quadriceps dominant.

If any of these muscles are tight or if you are quadriceps dominant, it will affect the function of your knee and potentially cause an injury down the road. Do the Knee Routine (page 146) to release the quadriceps and hip muscles.

Arthritis

The knee is one of the most common joints affected by wear and tear arthritis. Think about how many people you know over age 50 who have had a total knee replacement. Osteoarthritis happens when our joints are chronically overloaded, creating micro-traumas that accumulate over time. In short, the articular cartilage can't bear the persistently heavy load, and it starts to break down.

As you may recall from our earlier discussions, articular cartilage is the glistening white substance covering the ends of our bones that allows them to glide without friction. With no active blood supply, articular cartilage can't regenerate, which makes it particularly vulnerable to injury. Arthritis is the condition that occurs when this cartilage breaks down. Arthritis has many causes—from inflammation and everyday wear and tear to autoimmune disorders and bacterial infections. The solutions are as varied as the causes, but our focus here is on degenerative wear and tear arthritis, or osteoarthritis.

Degenerative osteoarthritis is multifactorial. Genetics, joint alignment, activity level, obesity, and lifestyle factors all play a role in joint deterioration. Of course, just like in the other areas of the musculoskeletal system, there are varying degrees of degradation that can occur. You can have mild breakdown and fibrillation, or at its absolute worst, the degeneration can be total—the articular cartilage wears off completely, leaving you with exposed bone, severe pain, and restricted mobility. That is termed bone-on-bone arthritis.

Any time you overload a joint, it puts additional mechanical stress on the bone directly supporting the articular cartilage. When our bone experiences extra stress, it increases bone formation, changing the stiffness of the bone directly underneath the cartilage, which causes the cartilage to soften. As the articular cartilage begins to break down, the cartilage's smooth surface transforms into what looks like a shag rug, and the tiny articular cartilage molecules break away and shed into the joint—a process called fibrillation. An inflammatory response to the damaged cartilage molecules causes the joints to swell, which makes the muscles fall asleep, and that forces the surrounding muscles to compensate, creating a whole array of potential imbalances. And while you can't feel pain in your articular cartilage—the blessing and curse of not having nerve endings there—you will certainly feel the swelling in your joints. Over time, the cartilage can completely erode and expose the bone.

At first, the cartilage is usually lost on just one side of the joint. And the beauty is that we can adapt and manage relatively pain free if we have normal cartilage on one side of the articulation. Usually with bone-on-bone arthritis, there is significant loss of joint mobility and, surprisingly, the swelling may start to dissipate. I believe this is because the joint cannot move as much and actually tries to fuse. There may be significant bony crepitation (popping, clicking, and crackling in the joint) as the joint surfaces move across one another, which has a distinct and often unpleasant feeling. The best way to know how much arthritic change you have in a joint is to get an X-ray.

Never Too Late

George, 72, is a fixture at my Toronto golf club and has been playing the game for more than 50 years. After his wife died, golf became the centre of his universe. Every day, he'd meet his friends for nine holes at 10:30 a.m. sharp.

One day as he was chasing a bad drive in the bunker, George felt a sudden pain in his left knee. George was terrified that he would no longer be able to play. George explained to me that he'd had intermittent knee pain and swelling for a few years. Every time the symptoms flared up, they would settle after a week of rest, ice, and gentle exercises. But it had never been worse than that. He had never blown out the knee on the course or shattered it on a ski hill. In the most recent flare-up, during that golf game, his leg was shot through with pain and felt like it might buckle. The pain receded after he did some physio exercises, and the joint never felt locked, as if it was blocked or stuck.

I took a look at his knee and leg. There was slight atrophying of his thigh and some mild tenderness along the front of the joint line, but the joint wasn't swollen. His ligaments were intact, and his range of motion was excellent. A knee X-ray revealed mild degenerative osteoarthritis. To me, this was great news. There were no signs of serious damage to the joint. The cartilage damage was somewhere between grade 1 and 2—far from the bone-on-bone scraping at the extreme end of the spectrum.

Knowing all this, I told George to follow the exercise routine I gave him and scribbled an additional prescription on a notepad: *Play golf.* I've never seen a bigger smile in my life.

George had been terrified that golf—a game that brought him so much joy—would be off limits. And for good reason: If you tell your doctor something hurts, they often tell you to stop doing it. My philosophy is different.

George's arthritis was from 70 years of wear and tear, his pain a signal that he was putting too much pressure on that part of the knee. What he needed to do was reduce the pressure to reduce the pain.

Because the issue wasn't structural, I looked for a source of movement dysfunction at his ankle and hip. Sure enough, George didn't have strong hip muscles, and his ankle was stiff. He could address these two areas with exercise, and that would significantly decrease the stress on his knee. George left my office with his "prescription," a list of exercises, and a big grin. I reminded him to keep moving and listen to the body's voice.

If you suffer from arthritis, you have to improve tissue pliability around the joint and improve the mobility and strength of the joints above and below. You also need to be patient, as it may take longer to achieve mobility goals if you have had arthritis for a long time. The body needs nine months to a year to remodel effectively.

Going Deeper

Damage to the meniscus in the knee can accelerate the degenerative process. The meniscus is C-shaped fibrocartilage that acts as a shock absorber, helping to stabilize the knee and dissipate joint loads. The outer third of the meniscus has a good blood supply, which means that there is the potential for a tear in that area to heal; the inner two-thirds have no blood supply.

There are different patterns of degenerative meniscus tearing. Most commonly, the meniscus tears slowly over time, progressively getting worse until a movement may cause the damaged meniscus to protrude between the moving joint surface and cause a painful catching or locking sensation.

This is an issue I saw with Joshua, a dentist who did his best to stay active, but with two young kids and a working partner, he found it hard. Joshua was bending down to give his young child a bath when he felt a sudden severe pain in his knee. His knee was so painful and became immediately swollen; he was not able to put any weight on his leg. Josh had to hand over the bath duties to his wife and head directly to Emergency, where the doctor thought he might have a meniscus tear. The ligaments appeared to be intact, and an X-ray showed no evidence of a fracture. There was tenderness on the joint line medially (inside of the knee).

Joshua was sent home on crutches and told to ice his knee. I saw him in the fracture clinic a few days later. His knee was so swollen he could not straighten it out. It was important to determine if his knee was locked because a fragment of the torn meniscus was trapped in the joint or if the limitation was due to the amount of swelling. Oftentimes people with a severely swollen knee lose the ability to contract the quadriceps. I encouraged Josh to activate the quadriceps and gently mobilize the joint to determine if his joint was mechanically locked. With coaching, he was able to extend his knee, so I knew the joint was not locked, and we confirmed a diagnosis of meniscus tear with an MRI. It is rare to have to perform surgery on meniscus tears. The key is to control the swelling, and the key to controlling the swelling is learning to activate your quadriceps muscle—see the Knee Routine for Acute Pain below (page 152).

Patients like Joshua, who have a degenerative meniscus tear without a locked knee, need to restore a Foundation for Movement at the hip, knee, and ankle. The latest research does not support the use of arthroscopy (minimally invasive joint surgery) to treat degenerative tears of the meniscus. The older you are and the more arthritis you have, the less beneficial arthroscopic surgery is in the management of a meniscus injury. In fact, the most recent literature examining the incidence of arthritis following partial meniscectomy suggests that patients who have surgery may develop arthritis faster. The jury is still out on this. My point here is that the path to recovery is unlikely to be surgical; instead, altering how you load your meniscus and knee can prevent the degenerative process from progressing. We know that people who tear their meniscus will develop arthritis 20 to 30 years down the road, so by changing how you load your knee, maybe you can extend that to 40 or even 50 years.

The second major structure of the knee that can accelerate the degenerative process if injured is the ligaments, most commonly, the ACL.

As you may recall from Chapter 1, ligaments are static structures that attach bone to bone, responsible for maintaining the normal anatomic relationship of the bones during motion—what we call joint stability. The ligaments act as check reins, preventing bones from moving beyond a specific range of motion to maintain normal alignment. There are four main ligaments that stabilize the knee: two collateral ligaments, which are on the outside of the knee, and two cruciate ligaments, which are inside the knee.

The collateral ligaments stabilize the joint to prevent side-to-side (varus or valgus) misalignment, while the cruciate ligaments prevent front-to-back (anterior or posterior) and rotational instability. Ligaments tend to tear because of sudden trauma, like a direct blow to the outside of the knee from wiping out at high speed while downhill skiing, not the accumulation of everyday wear and tear. There are some important exceptions, however, like the anterior cruciate ligament (ACL) in the knee. These ligaments can fail because of a sudden trauma, but there are subgroups of people—such as very flexible people and young female soccer and basketball players—who suffer chronic overload of these ligaments that results in tearing.

Interestingly, one-third of folks can function fine with a torn ACL. Another third can do some activities but no sports. And the final third has difficulty doing most activities. This is because of a combination of the alignment of the extremity, muscle-firing patterns, and the degree of stress applied to the joint, which depends on the kind of activities the person does. The ACL is essential for activities with sudden stops and starts and shifts in direction. For gentler activities, not so much. It is crucial that we maintain the normal alignment of our joints, one of the pillars for our movement foundation. If a ligament is injured and you do not compensate by improving dynamic stability of the joint, you are at increased risk of arthritis down the road.

Treating Arthritis

The key to managing and treating arthritis is focusing on what you can control. Unless you have a major operation, you can't control the static alignment of a joint. But you can control how you use your muscles (dynamic alignment), the kinds of activities you do, and even your diet.

Two and a half times our body weight transfers through our lower extremity with each step, so in some cases losing ten pounds of body mass can make a significant difference to the load on our knees. There is no shame in being whatever weight you are, but if you can change your lifestyle—how you move, sleep, and eat—and take some of the load off your knees, it may be a great help with any discomfort you're experiencing in your lower extremities. Muscles are your fuel-burning engines, and without them, your metabolism grinds to a halt. Increasing your activity can make a huge difference to your muscle mass. If you do decide to improve your diet, there's no question that it will positively influence your health, your healing, and your general susceptibility to any number of inflammatory conditions, including heart disease and Alzheimer's, as well as the pain you experience from osteoarthritis.

When it comes to the prevention or progression of arthritis, you need to understand your body. What triggers your joint pain? How much mechanical stress can your joints endure? How can you modify your movement and your activities so that you remain as pain free as possible?

Be smart and proactive. Control swelling, be consistent, and maintain your Foundation for Movement. You can live and move for a long time with abnormal joint surfaces. But if your arthritis becomes bone-on-bone severe or you're in constant pain, it's time to consider a joint replacement. That usually involves the surgeon removing the arthritic joint surface and replacing it with new metal and plastic parts.

While joint replacements can drastically improve your quality of life, they don't last forever. These new parts can loosen. And if they need to be replaced, you'll need a second, more complicated surgery, which brings risks like infection, dislocation, and post-operative blood clots. While complications are rare, they can happen. You need to weigh the risks and benefits. How much pain are you in? Can you sleep? Walk? Function? The more arthritis affects your life, the more worthwhile surgery is—but you need to be the one to decide. As a surgeon, I have seen the amazing benefits of joint replacement for the right patient. Even if you opt for surgery, it's essential to change how you move so you don't overload the joint replacement and wear it out in the same manner as the original joint.

There is good evidence that movement is medicine and that exercise can help ease arthritic pain. If your arthritis is so advanced that it is affecting the quality of your life, the benefits of surgery will exceed the risks. And if you've done the exercises, you will be well prepared for the operation and recover faster.

How Do You Keep Moving Even If It Hurts?

First of all, you need to address the pain. This means decreasing joint swelling and improving tissue pliability so that range of motion and joint alignment are maintained. By using my approach to release tight, non-pliable tissues with active self-myofascial release (ASMR) and isometric contractions, followed by activating the correct muscles, you will build mobility and strength around the injured joint.

By also improving the mobility and strength of the surrounding joints, you can allow inflammation and pain to settle in the affected joint. You can often progress with your activities as the improved function in the adjacent segments of your kinetic chain automatically take the pressure off the painful joint. I cannot emphasize enough how important it is to perform isometric contractions of all the muscles around the painful joint. This helps to control swelling, which will decrease pain and improve your range of motion. Understanding how much activity you can do before you aggravate the joint is important in the initial stages as you improve tissue pliability and reactivation patterns. I provide specific tips in the exercise routines below to help you decide when you're ready to progress to the next stage in your activity.

Anyone with knee pain should perform the assessments for the spine and hips (page 116) and for the foot and ankle (page 156).

Knee Routine

Restoring muscular balance, increasing tissue pliability, and improving movement and activation patterns at the knees and the areas above and below are critical for long-term resolution of achy and painful knees, and the Knee Routine does just that.

The first time you perform any new exercise, focus primarily on following the technique cues provided. Don't worry about counting reps. Once you feel you have a basic grasp of the exercise, start your first set slow and gradually increase how hard you contract your muscles. Work toward increasing your range of motion for the exercise. Rest for 30 to 60 seconds between each set and between exercises.

IF YOU DON'T HAVE KNEE PAIN: Cycle through the Knee Routine along with the other routines according to the Movement Longevity Schedule (page 196) that best accommodates your lifestyle.

IF YOU DO HAVE KNEE PAIN: If your pain is a 6 or lower on the NPRS, alternate the Knee Routine and the Ankle and Foot Routine daily for two to four weeks. Once you notice a significant decrease or complete elimination of pain, continue with a Movement Longevity Schedule. If your pain is at a 7 or higher on the NPRS, perform the Knee Routine for Acute Pain two to three times daily until the pain decreases to below 7, and then follow the guidelines above.

Quadriceps and IT Band Active Self-Myofascial Release

Releases tension and improves pliability of the quadriceps and IT band.

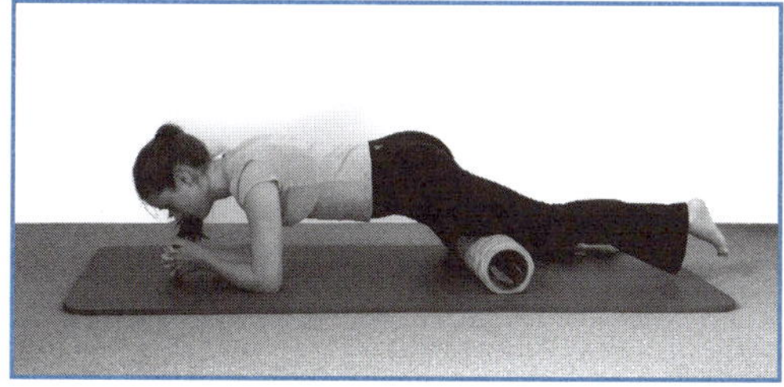

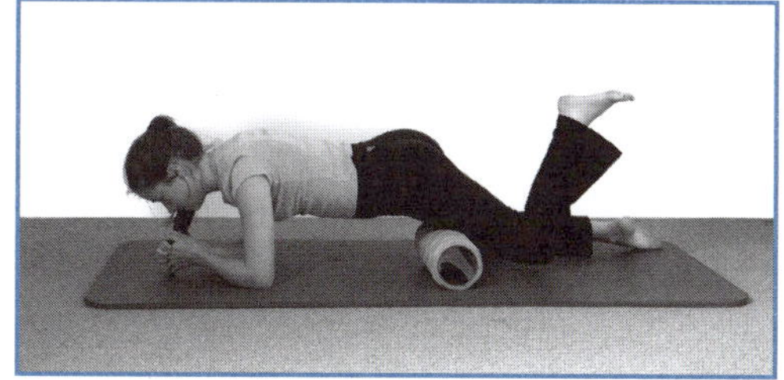

1. To treat the quadriceps, lie face down supporting yourself on your forearms or hands with a foam roller positioned just above one knee. Use your arms to walk the roller up your thigh toward your hip as you simultaneously bring your heel toward your butt.

2. When you reach your hip, reverse the motion to return to the starting position. Keep your thigh muscles as relaxed as possible so they "melt" over the roller. Continue rolling for one minute, varying the targeted areas slightly each time. Repeat on the opposite side.

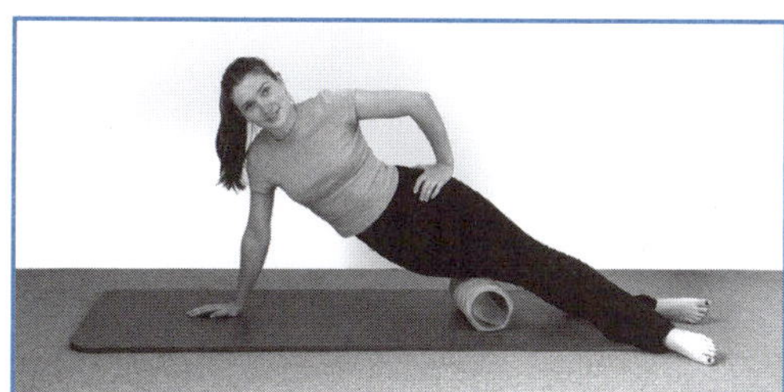

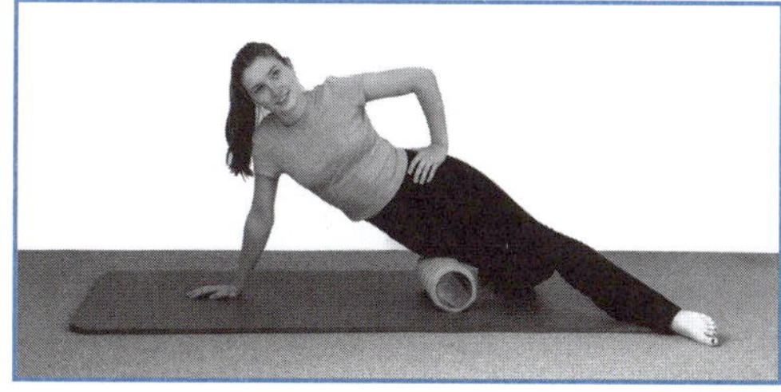

3. To treat the IT band, lie on your side supporting yourself with your hands and your top foot while your bottom leg rests on the foam roller positioned just above your knee. Use your arms to walk the roller up your thigh toward your hip as you simultaneously bring your heel toward your butt.

4. When you reach your hip, reverse the motion to return to the starting position. Keep your thigh muscles as relaxed as possible so they "melt" over the roller. Continue rolling for one minute, varying the targeted areas slightly each time. Repeat on the opposite side.

Extended Knee Ankle Flexion/Extension

Ensures all four heads of the quadriceps are working to provide stability and restore alignment to your knees.

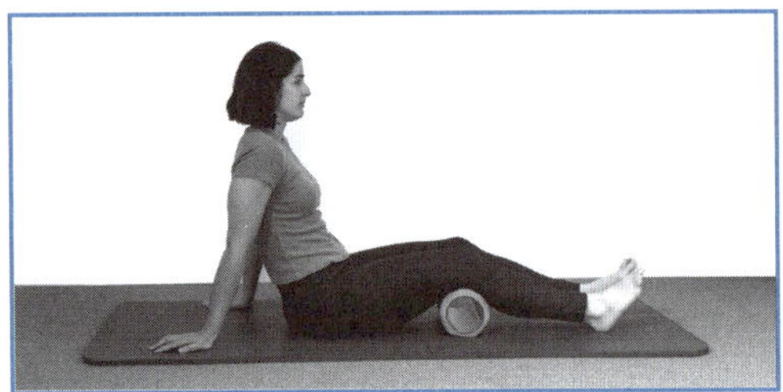

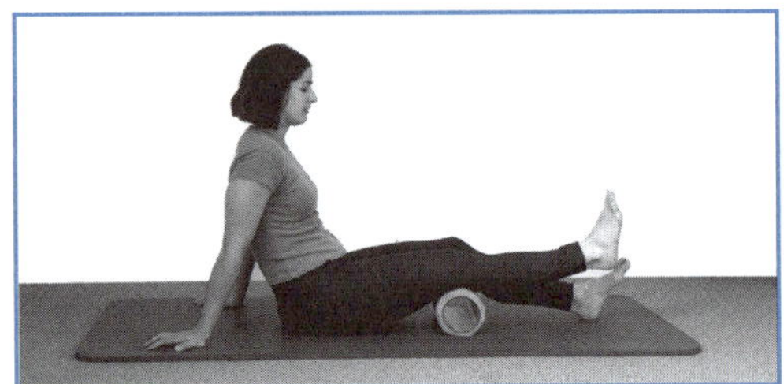

1. Sit on the floor, and place your right leg on a foam roller placed just above the back of your knee. Tap the muscle just above your knee on the inside of your thigh (the vastus medialis) a few times to wake it up.
2. Starting with your right heel on the ground, contract your quadriceps (the front of the thigh muscle group), and gradually increase the intensity to a strong contraction. Hold the contraction and slowly straighten your leg until it is fully extended, with your heel off the ground. Hold that position.

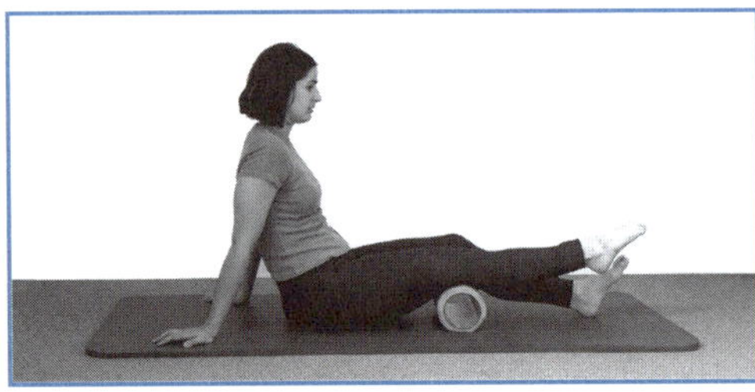

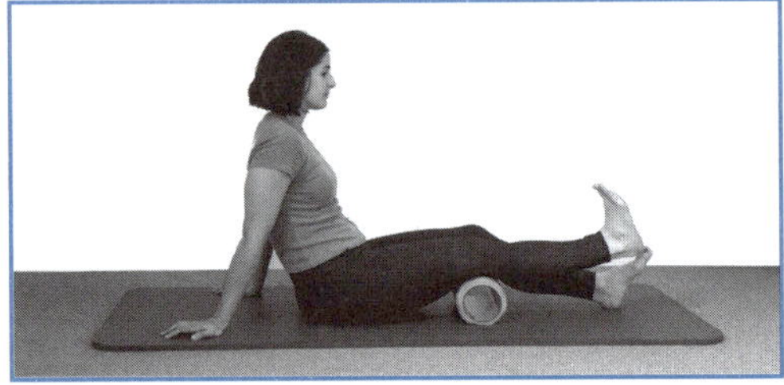

3. Keeping your right leg straight, contract your calf muscles (the back of your lower leg) to point your foot downward. Make sure your quad is still contracted as much as possible. Hold for five seconds.
4. Contract your shin muscles (the front of your lower leg) to pull your toes toward your knee. Hold for five seconds.
5. Return your ankle to neutral. Slowly lower your right foot to the ground. Gradually relax the quadriceps.
6. Repeat steps 2 to 5 eight times. Repeat on the opposite leg.

Hip Flexion End-Range Expansion

Increases hip flexion range of motion by strengthening the hip flexors and glutes.

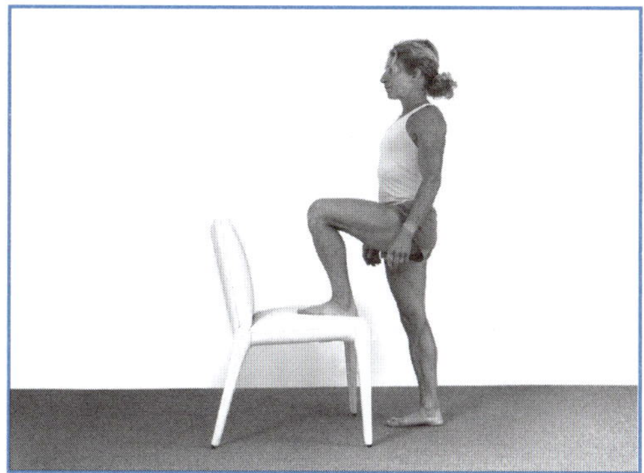

1. Stand tall and place your left foot on a stable surface with your hip flexed at approximately a 90-degree angle. Press your foot into the surface and hold for ten seconds.

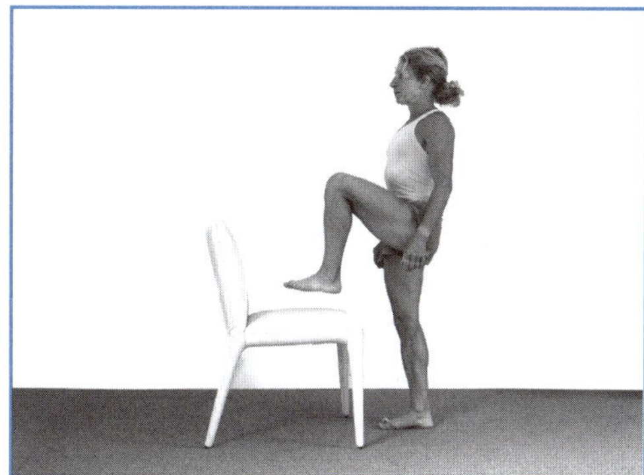

2. Maintaining your posture, lift your left foot as high as possible off the chair with a strong contraction of the muscles in the front of your hip. Hold for ten seconds.

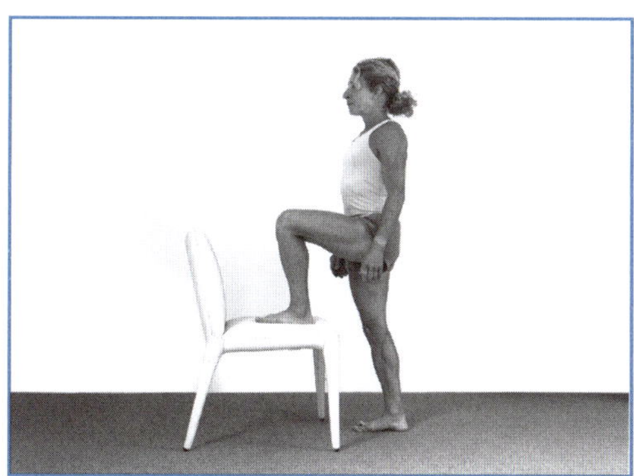

3. Lower your left foot to the surface, and then press it into the surface while contracting your glutes and maintaining your position. Hold for ten seconds.

4. Repeat the cycle three times, then repeat on the opposite leg.

Side-Lying Hip Extension End-Range Expansion

Increases hip extension range of motion by strengthening the glutes and hip flexors.

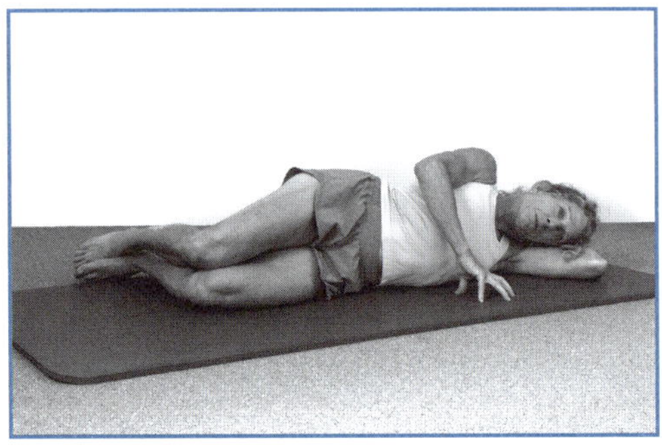

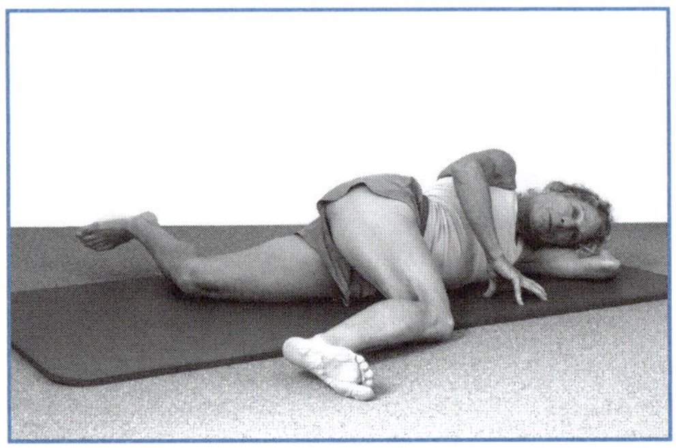

1. Lie on your side with your shoulders, hips, and knees stacked, and with knees bent to 90 degrees. Support your neck in neutral by resting it on your arm or a pillow.
2. Keeping the hip on the floor in position, flex your top hip to bring your knee forward so your thigh is at a 90-degree angle to your torso. Rest your top foot on the ground to stabilize your body. Contract your glutes as you try to reach the heel of your bottom foot farther behind you without tilting your pelvis or arching your back. Hold for ten seconds.

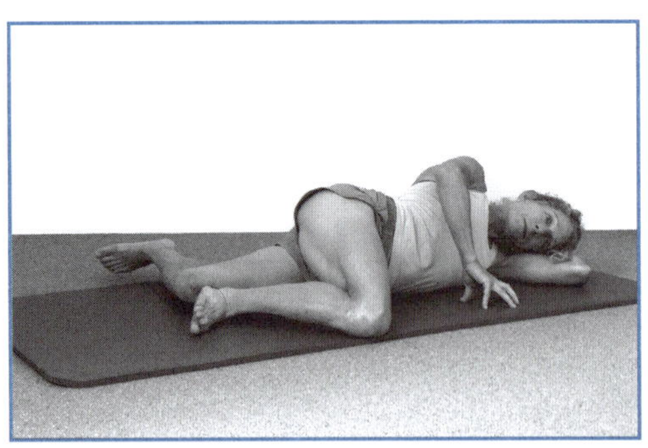

3. Touch the heel of your top foot to your bottom knee. Contract your hip flexors by driving your bottom knee into your foot for ten seconds. Your top foot should prevent your bottom leg from shifting forward during this contraction.
4. Repeat steps 2 to 3 three times. Repeat on the opposite side.

Standing Slumpy Psoas Activator

Builds functional strength in the hip flexors.

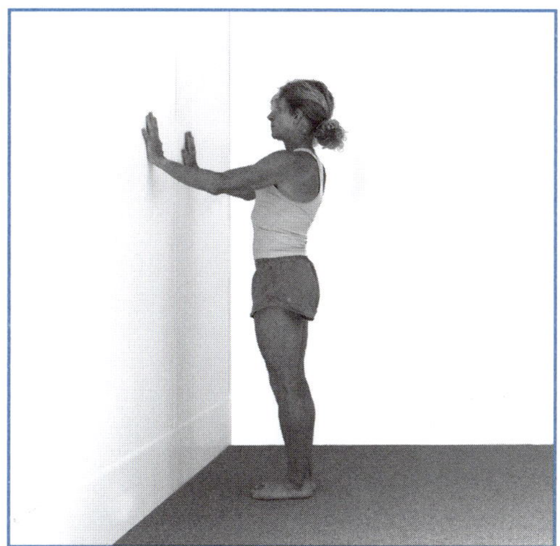

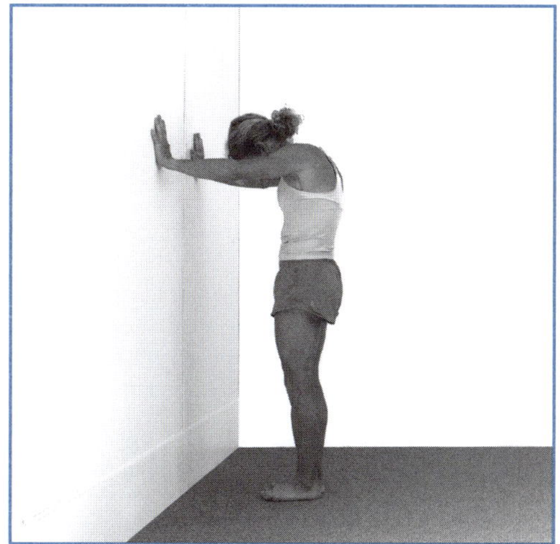

1. Stand facing a wall with your feet about two feet away from it. Support yourself by placing your hands on the wall, your arms straight out in front of you.
2. Get into poor posture: Curve your spine like a C, and tuck your pelvis under as though you are trying to tuck a tail between your legs.

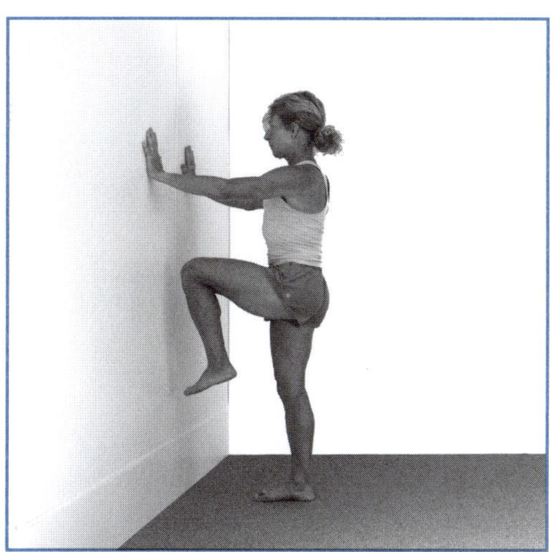

3. Contract the muscles in the front of your hip to lift one knee to a 90-degree angle. Simultaneously stand tall by straightening your spine and pulling your shoulders back. Hold for five seconds. Slowly return your foot to the ground.
4. Repeat steps 2 to 3 on the opposite side. Repeat ten times on each side.

Knee Routine for Acute Pain

If your knee pain is 7 or higher on the NPRS, start here. I used to have every one of my patients do this right after their knee scopes. Mobilizing the patella and doing isometric contractions will significantly decrease swelling and therefore pain in your knee.

Patellar Mobilization and Release

Decreases tension in the tissues surrounding the patella and can help decrease swelling.

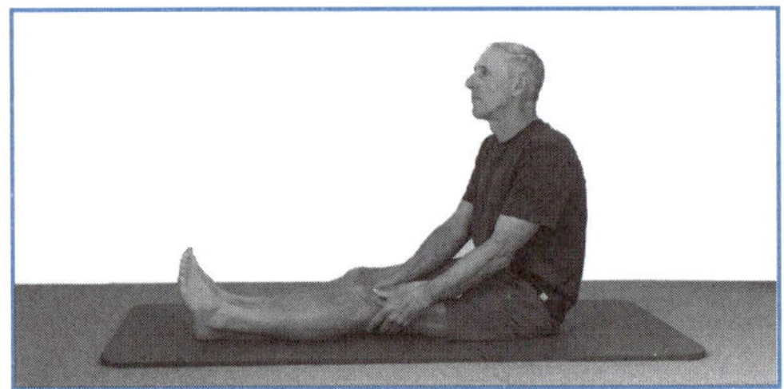

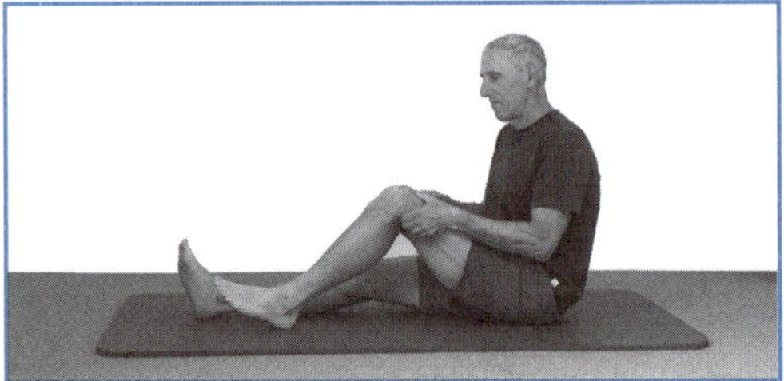

1. Sit on the floor with your legs out in front of you. If you have trouble getting up and down from the floor, sit on your bed instead. Work on one leg at a time. Place your thumbs on the top of your left kneecap (patella).
2. Bend your left leg while applying firm pressure and sliding your thumbs up toward your hip a couple of inches.
3. Repeat steps 1 to 2 for thirty seconds on each side.

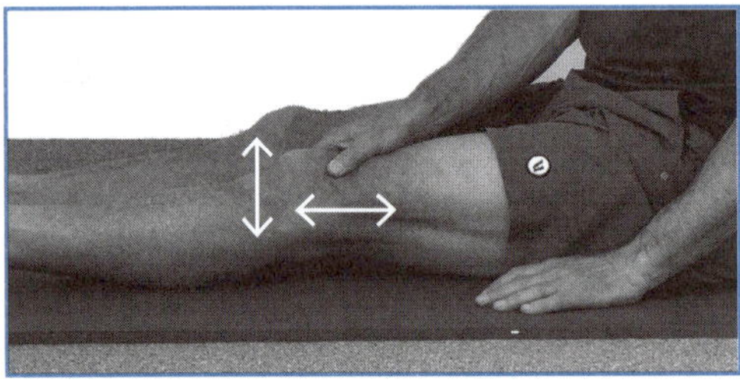

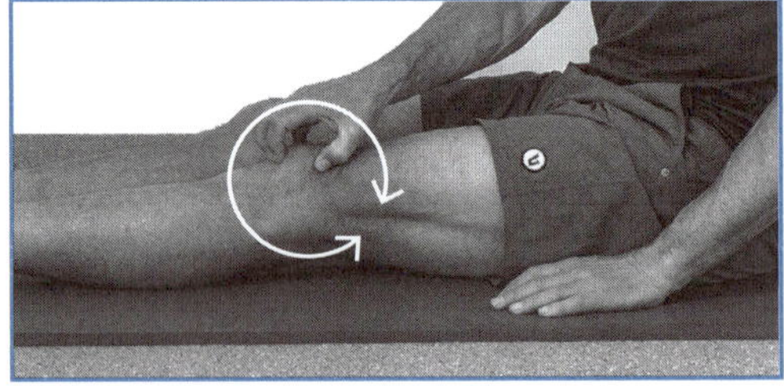

4. With your leg straight again, relax your quadriceps. Feel for your patella. Wrap your fingers and thumb around your patella. Slowly move your patella up and down, then side to side, for thirty seconds.
5. Slowly move your patella in circles for thirty seconds.
6. Repeat steps 4 to 5 on the other knee.

Quadriceps Ramping

Wakes up the quadriceps muscle group that often goes to sleep with knee pain and improves knee stability.

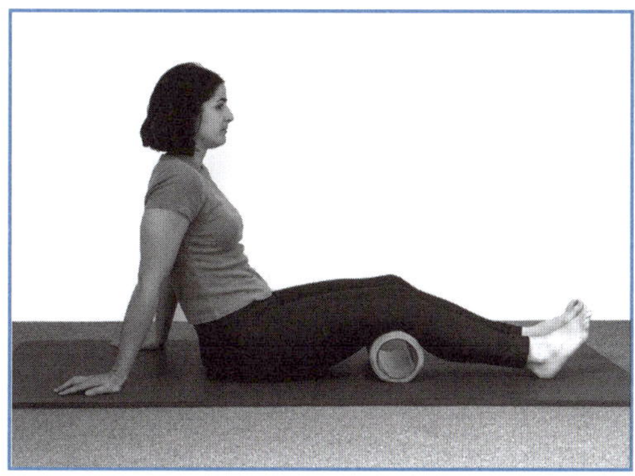

1. Sit on the floor with the back of your thigh resting on a foam roller or a firmly rolled-up bath towel so your knee is slightly bent.
2. Oftentimes the deep portion of the quadriceps (the intermedius) does not contract well. Focus on engaging the inside portion of the quad just above the knee. If you're having trouble, push your knee gently into the roller and scale back the intensity of the quad contraction until only the inside portion of the quad just above the knee contracts. You can also try rotating your whole leg toward the midline (internal rotation) to solve the problem. Activating the quad can take some time, so be patient.
3. Contract the quadriceps muscle by imagining you're lifting your foot off the ground, but don't actually lift the foot. Over the course of five seconds, gradually increase the intensity of the contraction as much as you can without any irritation or pain. Once you've reached your maximum intensity, hold it for ten seconds. Gradually relax the quadriceps over five seconds.
4. Repeat step 2 to complete five reps. Repeat on the opposite side.

CHAPTER 9

Ankles and Feet

The importance of our feet and how they interact with the ground cannot be overemphasized. Even though this is the last chapter focused on a key zone of the body, the foot needs to be addressed in every case I see. Almost every injury or wear and tear issue that we suffer starts in our feet. Our feet are our first contact with the ground, and if we do not have a strong and stable platform on which to move, we are doomed. If our feet—or even just one foot—fail us, then our Foundation for Movement fails us, and we will develop problems along the kinetic chain.

The greatest cause for a poor foot foundation is the shoe industry. I've heard some doctors and foot specialists refer to shoes as foot coffins; others call them sensory deprivation chambers. We are not born with shoes on, yet in large parts of industrialized society, we must follow the rules and wear shoes and boots. The result for many of us is that our feet have gone to sleep, and with them, many aspects of healthy movement have gone to sleep too.

It is amazing how much important sensory and critical motor input comes from our feet. Even though our feet are small relative to the rest of our body, there are 26 bones, 33 joints, and over 100 ligaments and muscles packed into them, and the amount of the brain's sensorimotor cortex that is dedicated to the feet is second only to the face and the hands. The sensorimotor cortex is the part of the brain that translates what we feel through our senses into bodily movements. Our feet are important for sensing information and then acting upon it. If you step on a hot stone, for example, you'll quickly feel the heat and step off in response. In addition to being a major source of sensory input, the foot has the same nerve roots supplying its muscles as our deep pelvic floor muscles, which form part of our core. Therefore, activation of the feet enhances the activation of our central core stabilizers. Our feet are supposed to provide us with key sensory and motor information to create a solid foundation for our kinetic chain. When they do not, there are consequences.

I was no exception. My feet were "dead": They were stiff, and the muscles no longer responded the way they should to maintain my Foundation for Movement. And guess what happened to me? Yep, more wear and tear injuries: plantar fasciitis, Achilles tendonitis, and ankle sprains, all of which could have been prevented by properly engaging and moving my feet and ankles.

DO YOU HAVE STIFF ANKLES AND SLEEPY FEET?

1. Test your ankle dorsiflexion. Start by kneeling with one knee on the ground and the opposite knee stacked directly above your ankle. Your front foot should be about a hand width away from a wall. Try to touch your front knee to the wall while keeping that foot perpendicular to the wall and its heel in contact with the ground. If you have a stiff ankle, you may try to compensate by twisting your hips, shifting your ankle off the perpendicular, or lifting your heel off the ground. Notice if you are trying to compensate. Does your knee touch the wall? If it does, congrats, you pass the ankle dorsiflexion test! This indicates good dorsiflexion for general movement. If it does not touch, you have work to do. Test both ankles.

2. Test your ability to activate the small muscles in your feet. Stand with your feet one fist width apart, your second toes facing forward. Test one foot at a time. With your weight evenly distributed across your feet, try to lift your big toe up while keeping the other four toes down. Don't let your weight shift to the big toe or little toes as you do this. Then try to keep the big toe down and lift the other four toes up. Again, hold even pressure across the foot while controlling your toe movements. If you cannot do this, do not worry; you can teach your toes to move again. Test both feet.

If you have a weak foundation in your ankles and feet, do the Ankle and Foot Routine (page 163).

Going Deeper

My lack of ankle dorsiflexion as an adult was most likely the result of inadequately rehabilitated ankle sprains combined with poor gluteal muscle function from lots of sitting and poor standing posture. Sometimes it is hard to know which comes first: poor foot function or poor gluteal function. If our feet are not working properly, we begin to use the muscles on the front of our body more, which is known as quadriceps dominance; we are made to use the back of our body for movement, to have gluteal dominance. If you look at anatomy books, the back of our body generally has bigger muscles and stronger sheets of fascia to transfer load from the ground up. A poor foot foundation has ramifications all the way up the kinetic chain.

Sprained ankles are as common as they come. They are often associated with an inversion injury (the foot rolls out), and they can happen when you land on someone else's foot after jumping up for a rebound playing basketball, or when you take an awkward step on an uneven surface. You might wind up twisting your ankle and tearing the ligaments that keep the ankle bones in place. The basketball injury is exactly what happened to me while playing in the provincial high school championships.

When it comes to an ankle sprain, there are three grades of severity. There are three ligaments that wrap around the outside of the ankle, and the grade of severity depends on the degree of tearing, which can range from a stretch to a complete tear, and the number of ligaments injured. The most commonly injured ligament is called the anterior talofibular ligament; it sits just in front of the outside bone called the fibula. The ligaments on the outside of the ankle prevent it from inverting, or "going over." In a more severe sprain, the injury extends from the front, around the side, and to the back of the ankle to affect more of the ligaments. The worst case is when all the ligaments that prevent inversion are torn.

With a low-grade injury, you may be able to get taped up and continue playing. If you have a significant tear, pain, swelling, and difficulty putting weight on it will start immediately. A ligament tear around the ankle bleeds, which can lead to profound swelling. Ice the ankle, and compress the area to decrease the zone of injury. Over the next five to seven days, a black line may develop along the outside of your foot. This is blood from the torn ligament that has settled as a result of gravity.

If you've sprained your ankle many times, you may not get as much swelling as you did the first time, because the ligament has already torn. Once you tear the ligaments in the ankle, you no longer have the same static stability because the ligament heals in a stretched position. This is why it is so important to improve the dynamic stability of your ankle and your foot foundation after you have experienced an ankle sprain. Because there are stretched static ligaments, the joint can lose its normal alignment if the muscles do not control the position of the foot and ankle.

The length of time it takes for the injury to resolve depends on the severity of the sprain. Typically, minor sprains take about one to three weeks to heal, and moderate sprains require three to six weeks. You can expect to be recovering for at least three months for a severe ankle injury. The initial treatment for all three is the same. In my experience, the priority is to control the swelling to prevent loss of ankle dorsiflexion. This is done using the traditional RICE technique—relative rest (use walking aids as needed), applying ice, compression, and elevation—and, most importantly, adding isometric contractions of the lower leg muscles to promote tissue remodelling. How long you spend working on your tissue quality depends on how severe the ligament injury is and how much swelling you develop.

OSTEOCHONDRITIS DISSECANS

If your ankle sprain isn't recovering normally, there could be damage to more than just the ligaments. Sometimes, the bone and cartilage in the joint also need to be repaired. Osteochondritis dissecans is a disorder that affects the bone directly below the cartilage. It is thought that trauma to the bone leads to the injury and death of bone cells in a part of the ankle known as the talus. Sometimes the injured bone can heal without any consequence, but other times, during the remodelling phase when the new bone is not as strong, the cartilage over the area can break off. This piece becomes a "loose body" and can get caught between the bones that form the ankle, causing a locking sensation, a feeling of giving way, swelling, and pain. If you are not recovering normally from an ankle sprain, get an X-ray to make sure you didn't damage the joint surface when you sprained your ankle. Sometimes, if the loose body is cartilage, you may not see it on a plain X-ray, so if there is swelling in the joint and ongoing pain that is not responding to treatment, you may need an MRI to confirm the diagnosis.

Rarely Too Late

The most common mistake people make following an ankle sprain is not fully committing to rehab. And because of that, either the ankle and foot stiffens or the muscles don't get strong enough to give the joint dynamic stability. It is important to regain proper mobility and strength to avoid further episodes of ankle instability, as well as other problems in the ankle region and up the kinetic chain. Research has shown that people who have suffered from recurrent ankle sprains are more prone to hamstring tears and knee pain.

When you have lost one of the static stabilizers for a joint, improve your dynamic stability to compensate. We do this by ensuring that all the muscles around the ankle and the foot—including the toes—are active, alert, and doing their jobs. We can train the skin to provide feedback on the position of the joint by using compression sleeves or kinesiology tape.

As with any other injury to the body, healing an ankle can be impeded by jumping up the Performance Pyramid too quickly and returning to your usual activities before you've achieved a good Foundation for Movement. On rare occasions, surgery is needed to remove a loose body, stimulate bone healing from osteochondritis dissecans, or tighten the ligaments around the joint. But even if you're going under the knife, you will get the best results post-surgery if you re-establish your Foundation for Movement pre-surgery. If your ankle is moving relatively well and the muscles are awake and ready to work once they are called upon, they will do their jobs and keep the joint aligned.

I did not regain proper ankle dorsiflexion after my ankle sprains, and I "got away with it" for years. Eventually, though, I suffered from Achilles tendonitis and plantar fasciitis partly because of the sprain and loss of dorsiflexion (from my failure to rehabilitate the ankle). The Achilles tendonitis arose when I was working at Sunnybrook Hospital in Toronto during my residency. It was slightly farther away from my home than my previous placement, so I was running more every day. Also, Sunnybrook is a very large hospital, set on 154 acres of land. It was a long way from the call room to the emergency room (although we were so busy, I rarely got there!). I am sure you can see the problem here: too much running, not enough recovering. My Achilles tendon was tearing more than it was repairing. I actually got to the point where I had a swelling in the centre of my tendon; the back of my ankle looked like a snake that had swallowed a mouse! I addressed the issue with a change in footwear, rest, and a slowdown in running. Things got better. In fact, the tendon completely remodelled, and the pain and swelling went away. With restored ankle dorsiflexion, my feel and ankles continue to feel great and I don't experience any more pain.

But the problem then seemed to transfer to my plantar fascia! The plantar fascia, a thick fascial structure running along the bottom of your feet, can tear much like a tendon. And when the plantar fascia is overloaded—often because of misalignment (e.g., flat feet or excessive supination)—and the glutes are inactive, the plantar fascia becomes overloaded and degenerates. The pain is usually right at the base of the heel. I don't have flat feet, but I had weak feet. The intrinsic muscles in my feet were not working well. There are very important muscles in the feet that when active act like little trampolines. Every step you take, they absorb force and send it up the kinetic chain. When these muscles are not working, the plantar fascia bears the brunt of every step we take. Eventually micro-tears are too numerous, and the body cannot keep up with the repairs of the fascia.

A damaged plantar fascia can be exquisitely painful first thing in the morning. Overnight, your body tries to repair the area, but it takes time for the repair to mature and for the tissues to become pliable, so as soon as you put weight on it, the vulnerable tissue starts to tear again. As with any tendon or fascial overload, we need to create a Foundation for Movement to allow the plantar fascia to heal. To speed up recovery, you can improve tissue pliability by (1) standing in a warm bath, (2) rolling your foot over a ball, and (3) activating your foot intrinsics. Warming up the tissues helps to ease the stress over the injured part of the fascia, protecting the overnight healing. Today, I'm able to maintain my pain-free status by doing the Ankle and Foot Routine at least once every week. These exercises will help you, too, establish a proper foot foundation, which will reset the neuromuscular system, restore balance to movement, and strengthen your foot and posterior chain muscles. And that will go a long way in taking the stress off your plantar fascia.

Long-Term Consequence of Improper Shoes or Unlucky Genetics?

When we wear shoes with a tight toe box, our feet get scrunched into a smaller space than they might like. A lot of the time, we wear uncomfortable shoes to look good or stay in fashion, but we need to be aware of the impact that shoes can have on the shape of our feet. There is a genetic component to the shape of our feet—some people are born with flatter feet, some with fatter feet, and some with crooked toes—but shoes have a massive impact on our function, mainly because they affect one of the pillars of our Foundation for Movement, the alignment of our feet. Changing the orientation of our feet with heel heights, the shape of the toe box, and even the amount of cushion can interfere with the normal activation (another pillar!) of our foot core. Those are the deep muscles in our feet that are so important for connecting the ground and our body, from the toes to the nose. This is not to suggest you should never wear a stylish but constraining shoe. But you should balance the amount of time in shoes with some good old-fashioned barefoot walking around the house, as well as exercises to maintain your foot foundation.

When Marla was 16 years old, she noticed that her big toe had become crooked; instead of pointing straight ahead, her big toe was aimed at her second toe. In doctor speak, we call this hallux valgus. She noticed that a painful bump was forming on the inside of her foot at the base of the big toe. It was red, tender, and making it hard to find comfortable shoes, let alone run and play sports! Marla had a hallux valgus deformity and as a result a bump, known as a bunion, was developing as well. The good news is that we could grab the big toe and straighten it out, indicating a flexible deformity with no major joint destruction, so her alignment could be corrected with exercise. The misaligned toe was created by improper balance of the muscles that normally move the toe. What would happen to a tent if the ropes on one side were too tight? The tent would begin to tilt toward the side of the tight ropes. Just like the tent ropes, all the little muscles in your feet work to maintain balance as they move the toes. If the ropes (muscles and tendons) are too tight on one side compared to the other, then the toes become misaligned. The solution, of course, is to balance the ropes, or the muscles, so that alignment is maintained.

We commonly see all kinds of different misalignment of the toes: claw toes, hammer toes, bunions, and mallet toes. Each of these deformities is due to a specific pattern of muscle imbalance. The solution in all cases is to awaken the feet with the routine on page 163 and, of course, have a good look at the shoes you wear.

If you did not come across this book soon enough and have suffered with painful toe deformities your whole life, it is possible that you will develop some arthritis in your foot. So long as the joints still move, I would encourage you to try to slowly get them going again. Your joints may feel like a rusty door hinge, so it may take some time, but don't give up on those stiff and tender tootsies. Every little bit of motion can help set you up for success. Our feet are great adaptors, so stiffness in one area can lead to more mobility in another. Strengthening the muscles to support the area that is compensating will serve you well.

I want to emphasize the importance of everyday actions that help your feet to sense your world and *wake up*. One of the best ways to activate the small muscles in your feet is to sit in the seiza position, a traditional Japanese posture. Begin by kneeling on the floor with your knees close together, and gently sit back on your heels, so that your buttocks are at or just above your heels. You can support yourself with your toes or place the tops of your feet on the ground with the toes touching, against your buttocks just resting on your calves and heels. You may not last long if you have been sitting in a chair for years like me. When I first started, I could only last 30 seconds before it was too painful. I not only felt pain in my knees but tight discomfort in my quads *and* my feet cramped. I was actually happy that my feet cramped, because a muscle that cramps is a muscle that can be strengthened! I tried to sit in the seiza position for 30 seconds three or four times per day. Gradually I increased to a minute, then two, and so on. Initially I also needed to do the following: (1) put pillows between my knees and feet to alleviate the pressure on my thighs and knees, and (2) place a rolled towel on the floor under my ankles. Decrease the size of the pillow and/or towel as your body remodels. It took me six months of slowly working at it to gain the ability to sit in seiza comfortably. Achieving a posture like this is an excellent goal to help you achieve foundational health. The beautiful thing is when you can sit like this, you know your feet, knees, hips, and spine are all in a better position and you are giving your fascia the chance to keep space for movement. Don't worry if you cannot adopt this position right now. Make it a goal to develop healthy postures to rest that help you maintain your range of motion and even create space in your body, including the seiza position, which promotes tissue regeneration. How we rest is how we regenerate!

Ankle and Foot Routine

The routine that follows will wake up sleepy foot muscles, restore proper foot and ankle range of motion, and give you the foundation you need to move with balance and grace.

The first time you perform any new exercise, focus primarily on following the technique cues provided. Don't worry so much about counting reps. Once you feel you have a basic grasp of the exercise, start your first set slow and gradually increase how hard you contract your muscles. Work toward increasing your range of motion for the exercise. Rest for 30 to 60 seconds between each set and between exercises.

IF YOU DON'T HAVE ANKLE OR FOOT PAIN: Cycle through the Ankle and Foot Routine along with the other routines according to the Movement Longevity Schedule (page 196) that best accommodates your lifestyle.

IF YOU DO HAVE ANKLE OR FOOT PAIN: If your pain is a 6 or lower on the NPRS, perform the Ankle and Foot Routine daily for two to four weeks. Once you notice a significant decrease or complete elimination of pain, continue with a Movement Longevity Schedule. If your pain is a 7 or higher on the NPRS, perform the Ankle and Foot Routine for Acute Pain exercises two to three times daily until the pain decreases to below 7, and then follow the guidelines above.

Plantar Fascia Active Self-Myofascial Release

Improves pliability of the plantar fascia and intrinsic foot muscles and mobilizes the joints of the foot. Progress this exercise to standing as your feet become accustomed to the pressure.

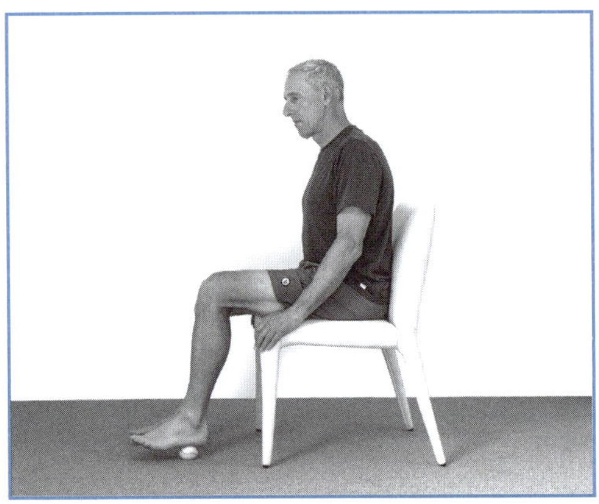

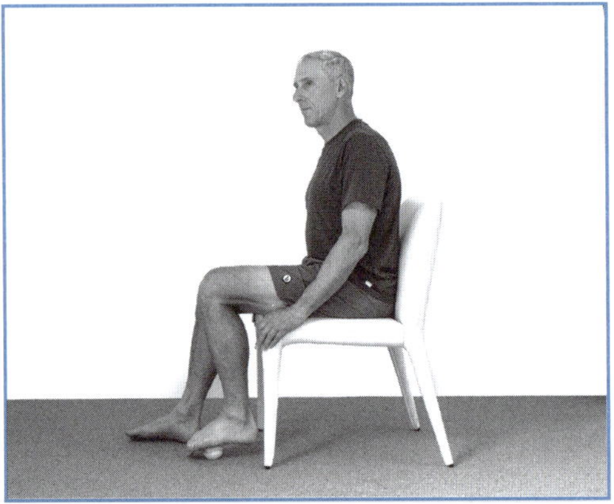

1. Sit on a chair and place your foot on a massage ball or other firm ball (e.g., a golf ball or baseball) with the ball just in front of your heel.
2. Maintaining firm pressure on the ball, roll your foot over the ball until it is under your forefoot while simultaneously curling your toes down. Roll it back toward your heel, as you extend and lift your toes toward your head.

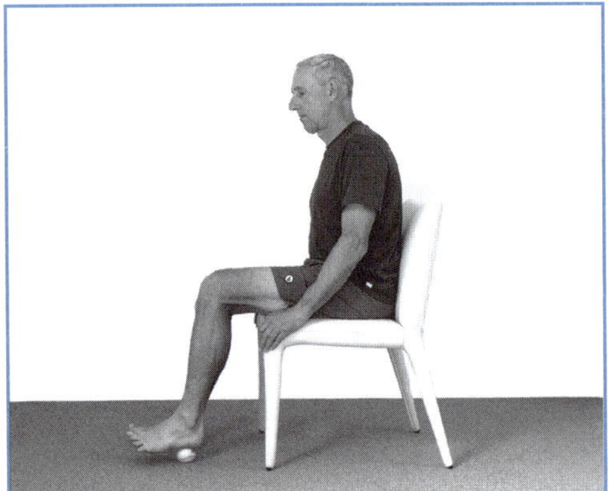

3. Return to the starting position, and repeat on different paths from your heel to forefoot for one minute.
4. Repeat with the other foot.

Short and Skinny Foot

Activates the all-important intrinsic foot muscles to create an active arch for better foot function and more efficient movement.

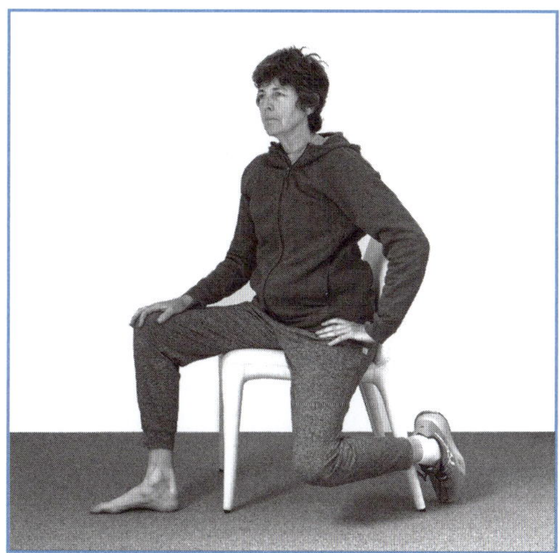

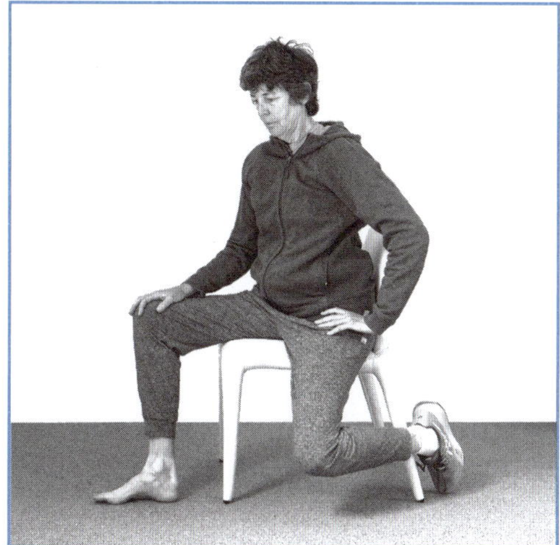

1. Use your fingers to spread the toes of one foot out wide. Keep a bit of your body weight on that foot.
2. Activate your muscles to make your foot as short and skinny as possible: Pull the forefoot toward your heel and squeeze your foot in across the forefoot. Do your best to avoid curling your toes. Hold for ten seconds. Relax.
3. Repeat steps 1 to 2 eight times on each foot. When you get more comfortable activating the muscles in your foot, you can exercise both feet at the same time.

Seated Tibial Rotations

Improves tibial rotation, a neglected range of motion, to keep your knees healthy, especially the meniscus and knee ligaments.

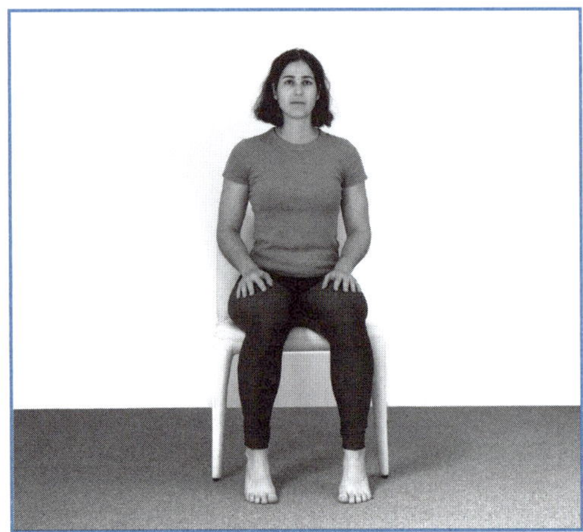

1. Sit on a firm surface that allows you to place both feet flat on the floor.

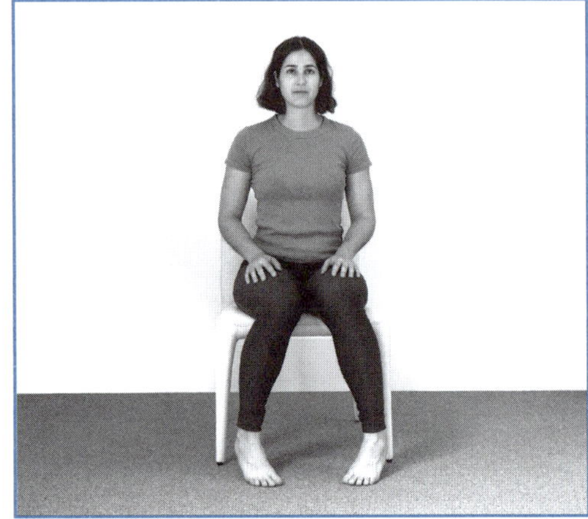

2. Doing your best not to let your knees cave in or move away from each other, lift your heels just off the floor and rotate them outward, holding for five seconds.

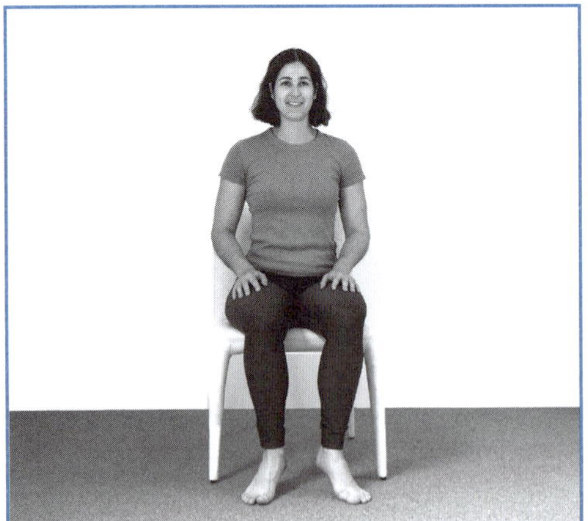

3. Rotate your heels inward and hold for five seconds, continuing to pay attention to your knee position.
4. Repeat eight times.

Ankle Dorsiflexion End-Range Expansion

Improves ankle dorsiflexion range of motion, which is critical for healthy feet, ankles, knees, and hips.

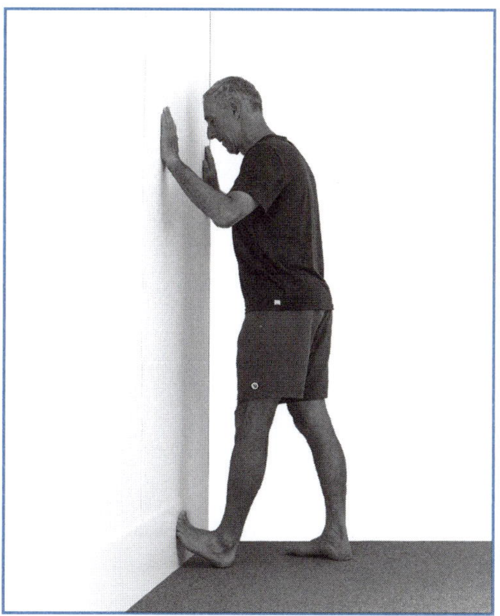

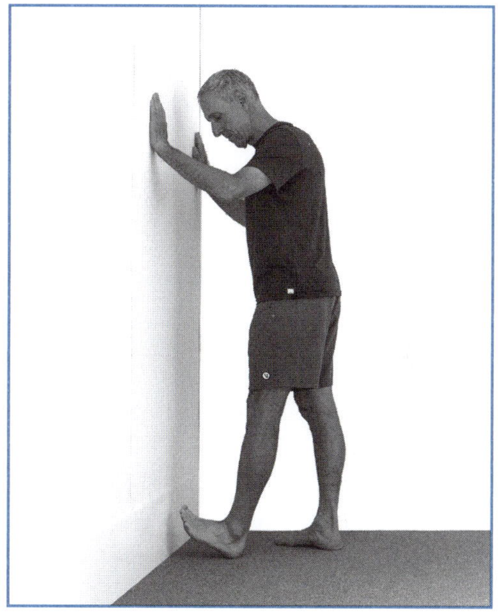

1. Stand in front of a wall, and place your foot on the wall so there is a very slight stretch of your calf muscles. Push your toes into the wall to maximize the stretch in your calf.
2. Lift your foot up off the wall using the muscles in the front of your shin. Hold for ten seconds.

Continues . . .

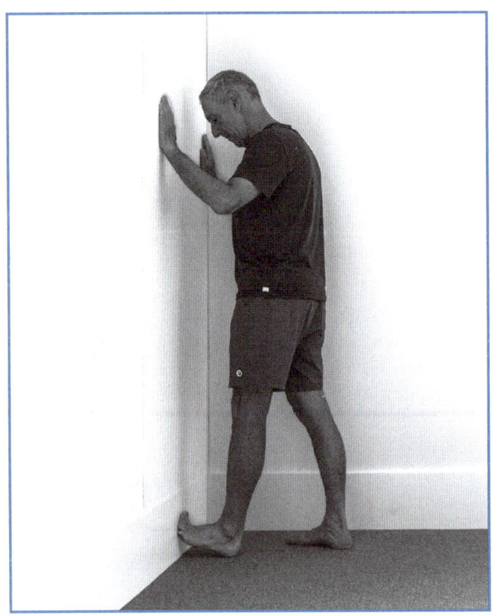

3. Return your foot to the wall, and press into the wall using your calf muscles for ten seconds.
4. Again, lift your foot up off the wall using the muscles in the front of your shin. Hold for ten seconds.
5. Repeat steps 1 to 4 on your other ankle. Repeat three times on each side.

Standing Glute Contraction

Wakes up deep muscles that contribute to the stability of the hips and pelvis.

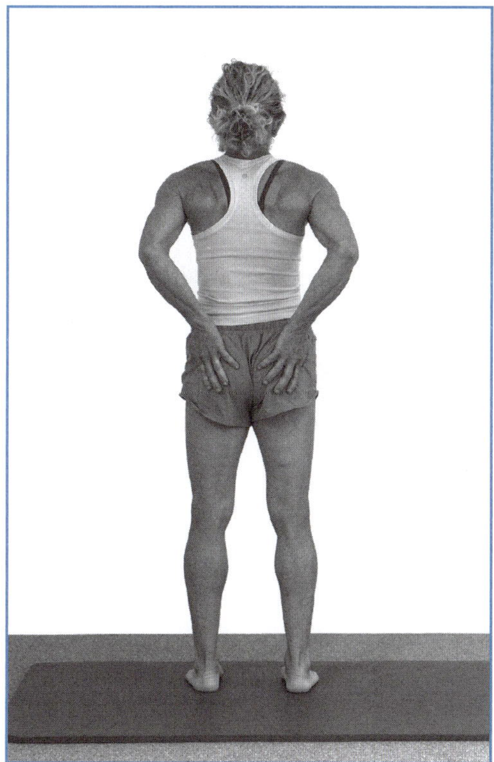

1. Stand with your feet hip width apart and pointing straight ahead.
2. Start with the Short and Skinny Foot exercise (page 165).
3. With your foot muscles contracted, contract your pelvic floor muscles by pretending to stop peeing midstream. Pull up and inward. Hold throughout the remaining steps.
4. Contract your glutes, ensuring your weight remains evenly distributed on your feet. Hold for ten seconds.
5. Gradually relax your muscles. Repeat five times.

Ankle and Foot Routine for Acute Pain

If your pain is a 7 or higher on the NPRS and/or you have any visible swelling in the foot or ankle, I suggest performing the Ankle Isometrics exercise (page 171) two to three times per day. I also recommend using ice up to four times per day, keeping your foot elevated whenever possible, and applying compression via a wrap to control the swelling. If you find walking painful or you walk with a significant limp, use crutches to avoid further irritating your already irritated body part.

Plantar Fascia Active Self-Myofascial Release *(page 164)*

Improves pliability of the plantar fascia and intrinsic foot muscles and mobilizes the joints of the foot.

Ankle Isometrics

Activates all of the muscles around the ankle to provide stability.

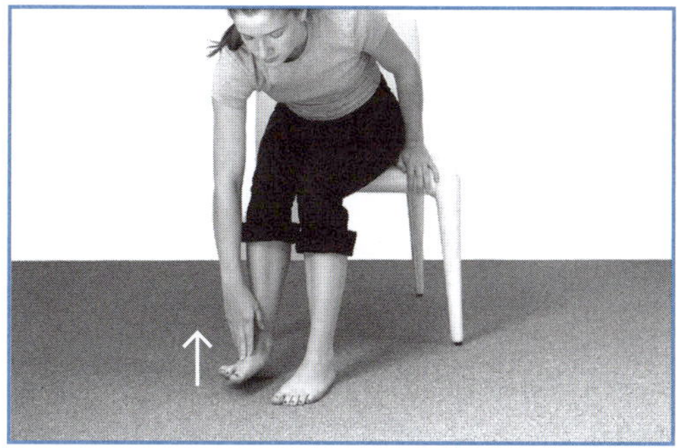

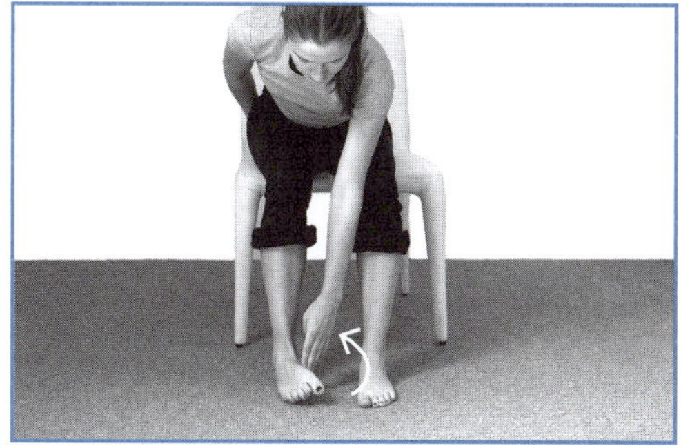

1. Sit on a chair with your feet flat on the ground. Apply pressure to the top of one foot with your hand to prevent movement. Gently lift the forefoot against your hand. Hold for five seconds. If you have trouble reaching your foot with your hand, use the opposite foot to hold it in place.

2. Shift your hand to the arch of your foot. Gently lift the middle part of your foot against your hand. Hold for five seconds.

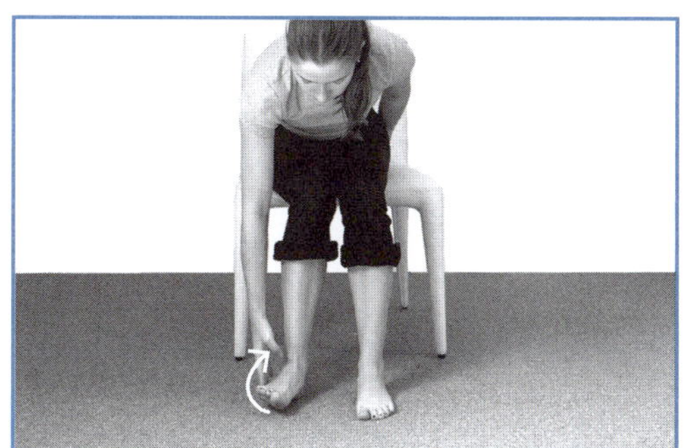

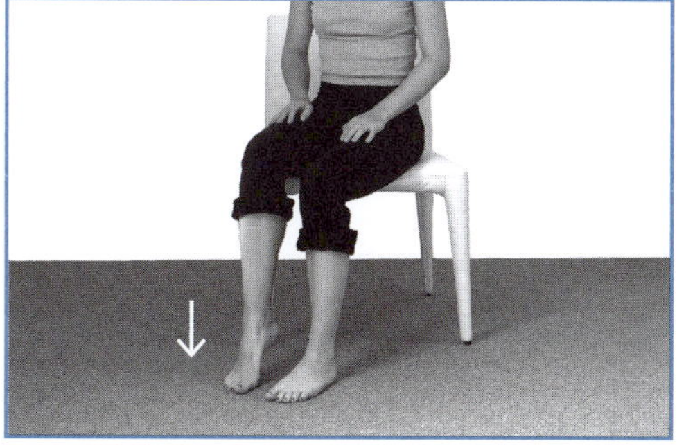

3. Place your hand on the outside of your foot. Gently lift the outside part of your foot against your hand. Hold for five seconds.

4. Gently press your foot into the floor as if you are pressing the gas pedal of a car. Hold for five seconds.

5. Repeat steps 1 to 4 three times.

PART III

Keep Moving Pain Free for Life

CHAPTER 10

Progressing Up the Performance Pyramid

After an injury, it can be hard to resist the urge to play your sport or get back to whatever activities you love before you're ready. It's not easy to sit on the sidelines and watch your friends play with their kids or feel like you need to ask your teenaged son to carry in the groceries.

Here's the problem: If you get back in the game before you're ready, you're going to hurt yourself again. The body needs time to heal, and the road to recovery isn't fast or easy. It's a process that requires knowledge, discipline, and commitment. It's a difficult tightrope to walk. Stay in bed all day, and your muscles will stiffen and atrophy. Push yourself too hard, and you'll make the injury even worse.

The Performance Pyramid can help guide you along that tightrope of recovery, carefully taking you step by step toward your goal, whether that's to finish at the top of your age group in the local marathon or walk your dog to the end of the street. The exercise routines in Chapters 5 to 9 are designed to help you re-establish your Foundation for Movement. Once you have a foundation, you can start to bring more endurance, strength, power, and speed to your movements. These are the key components of the Performance Pyramid, which will help make your body more resilient to the demands of daily life. If you progress up the Performance Pyramid carefully and incrementally while maintaining your foundation, you will keep moving pain free for life.

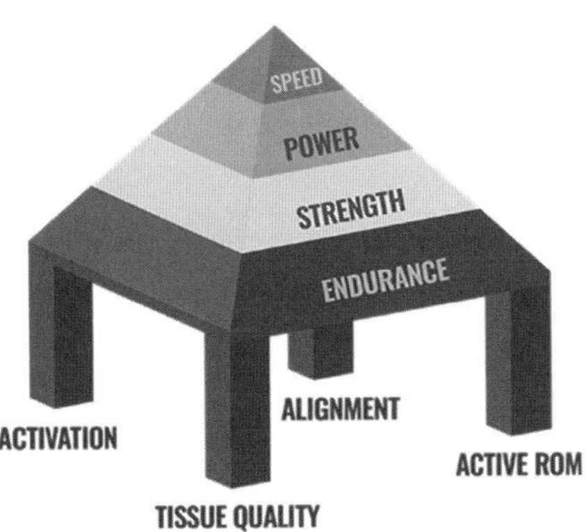

Understanding the Performance Pyramid

While working in the world of professional sport, I realized that most players with a significant injury struggled to return to their previous level of performance. A pitcher could throw again, but could he throw a 100-mile-per-hour fastball? I wondered why not, and from this question, I developed the Performance Pyramid to offer an approach to increasing and even maximizing performance in a safe way. The progression from endurance to strength to power and then to speed apply to any activity, whether that activity is something new we'd like to try or something we used to do and would like to get back to. As you climb the pyramid, it's important to remember that you can't skip a step, no matter how tempting. Like a house, you must build from the ground up. Otherwise, the whole thing will come crashing down. While our bodies may all be different, the principles of the Performance Pyramid apply to everyone.

Like building your Foundation for Movement, increasing performance is something that takes time. How much time depends on your body. If you have an imbalance in your hamstring that's developed over a few weeks of jogging, it shouldn't take long to get back on track. But if you shatter your knee in a nasty skiing accident, it could be months. The beauty of this system is that no matter how badly you may be suffering, or for how long, you can get moving safely and with purpose.

Setting a Goal

Before you begin making your way up the Performance Pyramid, it's helpful to know your endgame. What are you working toward? The needs of a pro football player are very different from those of a casual golfer or dog walker, so it's important to think about the particular demands of your activities. For instance, if you're a forward on a professional hockey team, you'll need a combination of aerobic and anaerobic fitness, as well as a fiercely strong lower body. If you're a marathoner, you don't need to be able to deadlift 200 kilograms, but you do need incredible endurance to make it to the end of the race. These principles apply to everyday activities as well. Your goal could be to climb to the top floor of your house or stand in the kitchen preparing food or clean the windows. Everyday life activities require different demands on our bodies, and we need to prepare our bodies for the heavy lifting in our home, work, and recreational worlds.

Your goal doesn't need to be extreme. Most of us just want to feel good. So whether you want to play golf again, walk the dog, work in your garden, or maintain independence to care for yourself, the way to reach your goal is the same: get moving, and keep moving.

Endurance

We have worked hard to establish our Foundation for Movement. Now it's time to build up our muscular and neuromuscular endurance, while maintaining the four pillars. Endurance ensures that the correct muscles remain active as we play our sport or perform our activity. This is especially important for newly activated muscles that have atrophied from lack of use and are prone to falling asleep.

During this phase, it's important to remember the little guys: the global stabilizing muscles. They're responsible for stabilizing your joints, so your bigger muscles can do the heavy lifting, and for aiding in the deceleration of those bigger muscles during hard and fast movements. If the stabilizers shut off, your other muscles will be forced to compensate, which not only impedes performance but also leads to more imbalances and injuries. It's equally important to focus on quality: It's better to complete a movement pattern once properly than repeat it multiple times with the wrong muscles.

But how exactly do we build our neuromuscular endurance? With three things: movement progressions, light resistance exercise, and cardiovascular exercise.

MOVEMENT PROGRESSIONS

It's important to feel connected to the activities you love, especially if you're still weeks away from being able to participate again. That's why I suggest using variations on the movements you would normally perform. Focus on rhythm—getting the correct muscles working together with the right sequencing and timing. This is what the exercises in Chapters 5 to 9 are designed to help you do. In the movement orchestra (page 16), all of the instruments must join into the movement song at the right time and intensity for a great performance. Start small, and work your way up with greater distance and intensity.

For instance, when it's time for spring cleaning, make a plan to do a little every day. If you have had a shoulder problem and are worried about reaching high shelves or cleaning the tub, plan to split the loads so that you reach for a high shelf on one day, see how you feel, and if you are fine the next day, do another. If you get sore, wait a day or two and focus on activities that don't hurt, and continue with your foundational shoulder routine. It will take longer to get the task done, but eventually your endurance and strength will get to the point that you can clean those shelves and the tub all in one day. As you're making your way through the Performance Pyramid, be keenly aware of maintaining your Foundation for Movement.

Movement progressions like this can be adapted for every daily activity and sport. Just remember that the movement must be a lighter variation of what you'd normally do. If you're a sprinter recovering from a knee injury, start with a light jog. If you are vacuuming the house, do a room rotation: living room Mondays, bedroom Tuesdays, basement Thursdays. If you're a golfer recovering from a back problem, try using just the short irons or even a half swing.

If you tend to use one side of your body repeatedly in your activities, you might want to consider trying to use your other side. Try brushing your teeth or your hair with your left arm (or right for you lefties). While you might end up with some toothpaste on your face, you're giving your right side some rest and challenging your brain with new patterns of movement.

The goal of this phase is to build endurance with the proper movement patterns to prepare you for the strengthening tier—and to have some fun.

LIGHT RESISTANCE EXERCISE

There's a time and place to find your one-rep bench press maximum, but the endurance phase isn't it. Although you certainly need a little strength to do even the simplest movements, the core of endurance training is high-repetition, low-intensity exercise. During this phase, I recommend practising body-weight exercises such as squats, lunges, and forearm planks alongside whatever skill-specific movements are required for your activities. You can build endurance by increasing the number of repetitions you do over time. Instead of just activating a muscular pattern, increasing your repetitions allows you to build endurance in the pattern. Losing your form is an indication that you are fatigued, and it's time to stop and recover. While increasing your repetitions, you need to be careful not to overdo it, especially if you're recovering from a serious injury.

Be sure to vary the kinds of exercises you're doing. If you're focusing on your legs one day (lunges and squats), you would benefit from switching it up and focusing on your arms or your core (planks and crunches) the following day. Not only does variety help you hit all the areas you need to, but it also means you're not repeating the same motion. Repetitive motion is often the very trap that causes imbalances in the first place.

As with movement progressions, it's important to start slowly. Remember pain is your body's voice, so if you're hurting after some light resistance work, you need to dial it back. However, if you wake up the day after a workout and you're feeling great, you can probably increase the intensity next session.

The same principle of simplicity applies to directional movement. You have to be pain free and stable in the frontal plane (moving forward, then backward) before you start moving side to side. Once you are stable moving in the frontal plane, add transverse side-to-side movements, and finally build in rotational movements to prepare for the return to your activity. Start with simple forward movements, like jogging. Once you're comfortable with that, you can move on to lateral movements, like side-to-side shuffles, and then rotational movements, like throwing and punching. Even in the grocery store, if you are recovering from a back issue, push your cart with your body well aligned with it, and when you reach to pick up something from high or low on a shelf, face the shelf and move in the frontal plane. As you start feeling stronger, you can begin to reach, twist, and rotate as you bend and lift your produce. Do things in a progressive fashion to preserve your Foundation for Movement.

CARDIO

Cardiovascular endurance may not be essential to your activity, but it is essential to the Performance Pyramid. When your heart rate rises, the blood flow to your musculoskeletal system increases, which brings more of the crucial nutrients necessary for healing and remodelling. The increased blood flow also allows your body to dispose of the waste that accrues in your musculoskeletal system during physical activity. What's more, cardio induces the development of new blood vessels in your musculoskeletal tissues.

It's important to get in a variety of cardio too. If you do the same motion over and over again, whether it's running, swimming, or cycling, imbalances develop from overuse. Switch things up! Instead of a bike ride, go for a swim. Instead of running, go for a bike ride. If you stimulate your musculoskeletal system in new ways, you'll build endurance *and* prevent further injury.

Strength

If you've built up your endurance and remained pain free with a full range of motion, it's time to progress to the strength phase. Unlike endurance, the core of strength training is high resistance and low repetition (two to six reps per exercise), and the goal is to get you stronger. With strength, you need to keep your endgame in mind. What kind of strength do you need, and what exercises will get you there? A quarterback doesn't need the strength and size of a linebacker, but he does need strong legs and a strong core to throw long bombs. So, as you're planning your program, make sure the majority of your training is activity-specific. If you're hoping to get out into the garden, make sure you focus on strengthening your core and legs so you can squat and pull those weeds without a second thought.

As in every phase of the pyramid, it's important not to rush things. You must be comfortable with the light resistance work in the endurance tier before you start going heavy with the machines or free weights. And if you have a choice between the two, go with the latter. While there is a time and a place for many of the machines at the gym, the problem is that they isolate one muscle, so you do not train the movement patterns of everyday life. The best kinds of strength-building exercises involve multichain movements that recruit several muscles at once, like deadlifts, an exercise in which you bend down and pick up a weight, using your glutes, hamstrings, and lower back. These kinds of exercises better mimic our everyday movements and require much more sophisticated neuromuscular coordination, a biomechanical ability that improves athletic performance and reduces the likelihood of injury.

Power

While strength is moving through resistance, power is moving through that resistance quickly. Strength enables you to lift a heavy weight. Power enables you to lift it in under a second. And like the strength phase, the power phase should be focused on specific activities and movements.

While power might be fundamental to professional athletes, not everyone needs it. If your goal is to play a casual round of golf, you can safely ignore this part of the Performance Pyramid. In fact, pursuing power generally might even be counter-productive, as it's the tier of the pyramid where you're most vulnerable to injury. But if power is crucial to your goal, go for it. Just tread carefully and remember to listen to your pain and watch for imbalances.

To cultivate power, focus on explosive but controlled movements. One of my favourites for tennis players is the box jump. To do it, place a sturdy and stable box in front of you. Then squat, jump up, and land with both feet on the box. Step off slowly and repeat. As you grow comfortable with the movement, you can increase the height of the box to keep challenging yourself.

You can also adjust the pace of strength exercises to make them power-focused. For instance, if you're performing a bench press, slowly lower the weight to your chest for a count of three seconds, and then explode upward as fast as you can. Just make sure you're nice and warm before you do this, or you might end up with an injury. And start with a lighter weight.

Speed

Once you've hit the speed tier of the pyramid, you should already be able to perform all the movements your activity demands. Speed just trains you to do it faster. Like power, speed is really only for those aspiring to peak performance. You don't need to run the 100-metre dash in under 15 seconds to be fit and healthy. However, for competitive activities, speed is almost always essential. In sports, it can mean the difference between winning and losing.

The kind of speed drills and exercises you need really depend on the sport you're playing. As a tennis player, most of the speed drills I do happen on the court, and they involve a lot of starting and stopping and lateral movement.

Balance and agility can be improved with ladder drills: Place a rope ladder on the ground and move through the rungs using different foot patterns. You don't need to be a professional athlete to benefit from these types of drills. If you don't have a ladder, you can use tape to create four squares (with 17-inch sides) on the floor. Practise walking on the balls of your feet by stepping into each square, one at a time. There are multiple variations you can create; for example, first move forward by stepping into each square with your right foot, then left, then alternate squares with your right and left feet, and finally walk sideways up the ladder leading with your right foot and then your left foot. Start by walking and then progress to running through the ladder, gradually increasing your speed. This will improve your reaction time and balance. I would highly recommend building these skills as they are key to preventing falls as we age. Regardless of what drill you're performing, build from the ground up. Start small and gradually increase the intensity. It's how we get better and how we prevent injury.

In training speed, one area athletes tend to neglect is deceleration (slowing your body down), which generally involves an eccentric contraction and requires significant baseline strength. Deceleration training is an important aspect of performance and often one of the first attributes to fail, which leads to the development of soft tissue imbalances and compensations. A strength and conditioning coach, if you have one, should incorporate exercises to train this aspect of your sport to prevent injury.

With all this said, it's impossible for me to prescribe a general program for power or speed. They're both too specialized and sport-specific. Strength, power, and speed are best trained under the guidance of a professional. They will not only help build a well-defined, goal-oriented program but also ensure you've got good technique while training. But if that's not an option, remember there are always ways to gradually improve.

Climbing to the Top

As you start ascending the pyramid, you'll discover that it isn't always a straight climb. Training for a return to your activity means fascia will tense, imbalances will return, and muscles will fall asleep. It's a never-ending balancing act that requires you to constantly maintain your foundation, even as you focus on moving up the tiers. As you move to the next level of the pyramid, muscles and neurological fatigue occurs, which may cause old patterns to return. No problem. Just do your routine to re-establish your foundation before you progress.

Before any activity, make sure your tissues are relaxed and balanced so that all the appropriate muscles can be activated. Practise the correct neuromuscular firing pattern before you perform your activity. Once you are ready, go and do what you love to do. It's possible that you will avoid developing imbalances again, but if you have had a chronic problem, more likely than not the imbalances will return until you have strengthened. So after your activity, re-establish the proper balance and activation pattern by spending some time firing the relevant muscles in the correct order. As you build endurance and strength, it will take longer for the imbalances to return. When you begin to feel really good, it is natural that you will push yourself longer and harder, so some imbalances and compensation can creep in. The key is to catch your compensation and correct it quickly.

Eventually, you will reach a point where you can incorporate your Movement Longevity Schedule (see page 196) into a warm-up as a prevention tool and performance enhancer two to three times a week instead of daily.

How do you know when it's time to move up to the next stage of the pyramid? First, you must be pain free and have a solid Foundation for Movement. You'll know the foundation is solid when you pass all of the foundation tests and are pain free. Second, your form should not be compromised at any point along the way. If you have faulty mechanics, you will be spinning your wheels, particularly if you try to progress to a more challenging phase of the pyramid. For example, if you don't use your legs when you're throwing a ball or lifting a heavy object, it will be hard on the rest of your body. If you aren't sure about your biomechanics, ask a professional, like a coach, physiotherapist, or trainer, to watch you so you keep your Foundation for Movement.

Other little things that can make a big difference include the equipment that you're using: Do you have the right racket, golf club, or baseball bat? The correct bike set-up or the right shoes? If you're not sure, check with someone who is. You don't want to do all this hard work to get back into the game only to be stuck on the sidelines because of faulty technique or the wrong equipment. And on the home front, wearing the right shoes and getting specialized tools and gadgets, like a lightweight vacuum, to help you through the rough spots can support your body for those daily necessities.

If you meet the two conditions above, you can likely take the next step. The ideal time frame differs for every individual, but six weeks at each tier—the time needed to make a big dent in neuromuscular development—is a good guideline.

Remember to monitor your NPRS, which we introduced in Chapter 2. Rate your pain on a scale of 1 to 10 before and after your workout. If you hit a high number (7–10), there are routines for acute pain in Chapters 5 to 9 that are very helpful. If you are regularly at a high number, you need to follow up with your doctor to figure out what needs to change. The beauty of the NPRS is you can follow trends, so observing your pain going from 3 to 0 is a great indication that you have found the right rhythm of recovery. If you observe your pain scale rising as you increase the intensity or duration of your activities, that is a clue that you need to back off a bit. Go back to the activity level where you were stable, and you should see a decrease in the number before increasing your intensity again.

Staying on Top

In my practice, I saw countless people progress through the pyramid and return to their activity only to come back to me a couple of years later complaining of pain. I asked each one the same question: "Have you continued maintaining your Foundation for Movement?" Each one gave me the same answer: "No."

The Foundation for Movement *and* the Performance Pyramid are how you stay at the top. They must be used together. Even with the best habits, our musculoskeletal system is not immune to tension, imbalances, and inactive muscles. These things are going to happen when you are active. To maintain your endurance, strength, power, and speed, you must put in the maintenance work, and that means identifying imbalances and adaptive movements so that you can reprogram them on a regular basis.

MOVEMENT MESSAGES

- Progress up the pyramid slowly. Crawl before you walk, and walk before you run.
- Use the exercise routines in this book as a warm-up or cool-down to maintain your Foundation for Movement.
- Track your pain using the numeric pain rating scale (NPRS) to help you decide when it is time to progress up the pyramid.
- Returning to an earlier phase of the pyramid is not a failure; it simply means your body needs more time to adapt. Give yourself that time, and then keep moving!

CHAPTER 11

Healthy Habits for Movement Longevity

I have always loved sports and being active, and I have had just about every possible movement dysfunction and wear and tear injury you can imagine. To this day, if I don't pay attention to my Foundation for Movement, I lose it. It seems that I always have a little something that hurts. As frustrating as this may seem, I view it as a gift. As I learn more about my own body, what makes it feel better or worse, and what accelerates my recovery, the more I can share with others.

Playing tennis not only keeps my body young, it provides me with feelings of general well-being and accomplishment, not to mention serious health benefits like lessening the risk of cancer, diabetes, dementia, heart disease, and stroke. I am moving better now than I did five years ago and even better than I did six months ago. My goal is to be running on the tennis court, playing games, and visiting my friends around the world when I am 100 years old. If you are not where you want to be, know that the time you put in now will pay dividends in the coming years.

Though it's not easy, there are many reasons we should give our bodies some love every day. To keep my musculoskeletal system healthy, I must give it some time each day. How much time? That depends on whether I want to head to the tennis court, walk to the grocery store, or walk around the block. To guide you in establishing healthy habits, I am going to share some tips that can act as a framework to help you develop your own system. It requires hard work to get in shape, but it takes very little work to stay in shape. Once you get going, try to keep going. The momentum it takes to maintain a good habit is far less than the momentum required to change a habit in the first place.

1. Practice the Four Ps: Prioritize, Plan, Presence, People

PRIORITIZE

Make your body a priority: There is only so much time in the day, and doing exercises like the ones shared in this book may be lowest on a very long list for many people. Exercise may come dead last to kids, work, friends, social time, running errands, watching television—the list goes on. The reality is if you don't make your body a priority, nobody else will.

I wrestled with this when my children were young. I remember them complaining when I went to play tennis on the weekend. I had to point out there were 24 hours in the day, and I was gone for maybe two. That left 22 hours with them! My body felt better, and I gained all the benefits that come with exercise: the endorphins, friendship, and good general health. I was also being a good role model for my children, teaching them the importance of taking care of their bodies and their health. And if I didn't take care of myself, I wouldn't be able to take care of my kids.

Fast-forward 20 years. Both of my children are active and work out regularly, and we all have fun playing sports together, going for walks, and then relaxing by watching movies and having a laugh. Activities and sports have given us not only great physical health but also a bond—experiences we can share and activities we can do together. I look forward to teaching my grandchildren how to play tennis, taking them for walks, and playing in the park. The things you do together build relationships and connection.

If your life is so busy that you can't imagine how you'll carve out time for exercise, you might want to start by walking up the stairs instead of taking the escalator when given the option. I used to intentionally park my car farther away from my destination. When you're standing in line at the bank or maybe watching your kids play sports, try moving around, contracting your glutes, or doing some of the exercises for shoulder mobility (page 101). Between meetings at work, you may have time to answer a phone call, grab a snack, and do a three-minute exercise to activate you psoas muscles (page 129). When we are physically strong, we feel mentally strong. Your mind and body need to be a priority.

PLAN

Write a daily movement routine into your schedule. I was a single mom with two kids under the age of four, running a full-time research lab and a clinical orthopaedic surgery practice, but I made movement a priority, and I did it by writing it into my schedule. When it was written in my schedule, it was written in stone.

Just as we might schedule a dental appointment or a hair appointment, I make a musculoskeletal health appointment: 20 to 90 minutes often early in the day, so I can get my endorphins going and my mind and body ready for a great day ahead. And as schedules can often be unpredictable, derailing our movement routine, it's a good idea to fit it in early before the day gets away from us.

There are so many positive side effects of completing your movement routine, including a sense of well-being, accomplishment, and pride in taking care of yourself. There are times in your life when you may be able to spare only a few minutes, but a few minutes is better than no minutes. Start small. Do one exercise each day and try to increase this to three, four, or five per day. Consistency is key. The more comfortable and familiar you become with the exercises, the more creative you can become about when and where you plan to do them. If it is impossible to get 15 minutes to yourself to do your routine, then you can contract your glutes or activate your foot intrinsics while sitting in a movie theatre or standing at a party chatting. No one else will know, but your body will! Give yourself the gift of mobility. Even five minutes a day will pay dividends.

The amount of time you spend moving may change over your lifetime depending on where you are in your career. Wherever you are, focus on your priorities and find ways to plan your day around them.

CREATIVE WAYS TO COMBINE MOVEMENT STRATEGIES WITH EVERYDAY TASKS

- While talking on the phone, do a variation of the Slumpy Serratus Activator on page 102 by moving just your shoulder blades while your arms rest in place.
- Perform glute contractions (a variation of the exercise on page 131) while sitting at your desk.

- Do chin tucks (a variation of the exercise on page 86) while standing at the sink washing dishes or brushing your teeth.
- When you're in the car stopped in traffic, do one Extended Elbow Wrist Fan (page 106).
- When you're stuck in a long meeting, practise a Short and Skinny Foot (page 165) in your shoe, or even better, take off your shoe under the desk and do it in your socks.
- While you're sitting watching television, perform two reps of the Slumpy Psoas Activator (page 129).

PRESENCE

Hopefully, you will reach a point in life when you have 15 minutes every day dedicated to your Foundation for Movement routines. If you need to squeeze in your exercises while you're watching your daughter's soccer game, that's okay, but whenever possible, be there and nowhere else. Enjoy the time you're taking for yourself. Connect with your body, and get to know it better.

Being present in whatever activity we are doing is a skill that transfers into every part of our lives, giving us better focus, better connections, better relationships, and a general feeling of well-being. Using exercise as a way to connect with your body—becoming aware of your breath and your limbs moving, the sensations of pressure, and the release of tension as you move—is an amazing way of connecting to yourself.

Especially when you're starting out, focus on your form. Do you need to adjust how you are performing the exercise, or do you have good technique? Notice how your muscles feel when they start to fatigue, and what your range of motion is. Become aware of your heart rate and your breathing—is it deep or shallow? Engage in the activity, and find moments when you focus, trying not to let your mind wander. It will go a long way.

PEOPLE

We need community. People support us in our careers, family lives, and recreational pursuits. They can support our movement goals too. Talking with others about how they exercise can be very illuminating. Asking for support if you need it at home or at work can give you the opportunity to take care of your body. Connecting with others through movement—with a team sport, through gardening, or dog walking—can be a wonderful experience. Finding someone or several people to go on a movement journey with you is fun, and setting shared goals with another person can help to keep you accountable. We all want to be connected, and it is helpful to be around like-minded individuals who can help us get where we want to go.

2. Warm Up and Cool Down

Many people can't be bothered with a proper warm-up, and it always seems to be the first thing to go when you're pressed for time. But I'm going to give you some advice: DO NOT SKIP YOUR WARM-UP. Think of your body as a car in the dead of winter. If you turn the ignition and just start gunning it, there's going to be a problem.

FIFA, the international governing body of soccer, developed the 11+, a complete warm-up program consisting of 15 exercises designed to reduce injuries among amateur players. They found teams who performed the warm-up at least twice a week had 30 to 50 percent fewer injured players. Better yet, the warm-up improved performance too.

What makes a good warm-up? It needs to do three things: elevate your heart rate, warm up your muscles, and fire up your neuromuscular system. Your warm-up should help establish your Foundation for Movement. So, if the back of your shoulder is a little tight, do some active self-myofascial release (ASMR) to balance it out, follow that up with a dissociation technique to make sure the correct muscles are turned on, and get those last few degrees of motion with an end-range expansion (ERE) shoulder sequence. Not only will you prevent injury, you will perform better. If you want to move forever and prevent injury, do a 5–15 minute warm-up before you play.

Doing a proper cool-down is important too. During practice and play, you become fatigued, and imbalances begin to set in. Cool-downs begin to resolve those imbalances and start your recovery off right. Remember that a natural consequence of movement is to lose our Foundation for Movement, so re-establishing the foundation as soon as possible will prevent us from losing our rhythm of recovery. When we recover well, we don't get injured. Time is a factor, so do your best to do it as soon as you're done moving. As long as you warm up well, you can get away with less of a cool-down, but ideally you should do both.

After a tough workout, I recommend 10 to 20 minutes of active recovery, like some easy spinning on a stationary bike or a brisk walk. Some light motion will help purge all the metabolic by-products from your body. I often walk my dog as a form of recovery. Next, follow up with whatever program you need to address your specific imbalances to reactivate any sleeping muscles and maybe some foam rolling. The beauty of establishing a good Foundation for Movement is that you don't have to spend as much time rebalancing and reactivating. If you're not sure what area of your body to address, retake the screening tests of the different zones of your body to check in on your foundation. This will identify any areas where you are lacking mobility or strength.

3. Switch It Up

If you perform the same motion over and over again, two things happen. First, imbalances develop from overuse, and second, the musculoskeletal system adapts to whatever movement you are doing, so your strength, flexibility, and endurance plateau.

Thankfully, there's an easy solution: Switch things up! This could be something as simple as trying something new. Instead of biking, go for a swim. Instead of running, go for a bike ride. You can also change the kinds of motion you're doing during your activity. For example, if you're a weightlifter who likes to go hard and heavy, try a session with lighter weights and change the speed of your workout. Try a different position on your team sport. In everyday life, instead of convening in a boardroom, go for a walking meeting, or ditch your chair and sit on the floor (great for squat practice). When we stimulate our musculoskeletal system in new ways, the body is forced to adapt. So whatever you do, it's good to keep your body guessing.

4. Allow Yourself to Recover: Follow the Five Rs

A great recovery begins with a great cool-down, but that's not where it ends. For your body to properly recuperate after a tough practice or a gruelling workout, you need to follow the five Rs of recovery: rest, rehydrate, refuel, regenerate, and relax. Make recovery part of your daily routine.

REST

Our body repairs the day's micro-injuries as we rest. If you don't rest or get enough sleep, you're not giving the body enough time to repair the day's damage, making you vulnerable to a wear and tear injury. While each person's body is different, aim for at least eight hours of sound sleep every night.

Remember that our bodies respond to the physical stresses applied to it. Not only when we are moving, but when we are resting, these forces cause our connective tissues to remodel. How we rest is how we heal. If we sit for hours in a slouched position on the couch, on our computers, or in the car, our fascial system remodels to that shape. We will be fighting a losing battle if we exercise for a short period of time and then sit or stand still for the remainder of our day in a posture that does not promote our foundation. Use your rest time to promote the maintenance of your foundation. I recommend adopting the postures of children and Indigenous cultures, where chairs and cars are often not used. Sit on the floor, cross-legged, or in the seiza position (see page 162). If you have not sat in these positions for years, they will be challenging, but you will not believe how good you feel after using them regularly for a month. Try sitting on the floor for 30 seconds three times per day, and over a month or two, work your way to the point that you can sit and eat lunch on the floor. If you need to use pillows to support your knees and spine in good alignment, use them. How you rest will help determine how you heal, and resting well makes it so much easier to maintain your Foundation for Movement.

REHYDRATE

It should go without saying that good health requires good hydration. Drinking enough water is absolutely essential to recovery. Drink half an ounce for every pound you weigh (or approximately 30 millilitres per kilogram). A 150-pound person should drink 75 ounces of water per day. If you are working out and sweating a lot, you'll need to drink even more. I would recommend adding electrolytes to your water in this situation.

REFUEL

The body needs raw materials to make its repairs, and those raw materials come from a healthy, well-balanced diet. Without proper nutrition, the body will rob Peter to pay Paul, stealing repair molecules from existing muscle to repair the day's micro-injuries, thereby preventing new muscle growth. The timing of your food intake is important too. To maximize recovery, you should provide your body with some glucose and protein within 30 minutes of exercise.

REGENERATE

Give your body the time it needs to regenerate and repair. Once you're properly rested, rehydrated, and refuelled, your body can begin to regenerate. How much time you need to regenerate depends on a number of factors, ranging from the intensity of your workout to your emotional state. Pay attention to your body, and be sure you're properly recovered before your next training session. Give your body the time to heal.

RELAX

The body and the mind are so interdependent that tension in one causes tension in the other. Learning how to relax both is crucial to maintaining pain-free movement. While relaxing the mind and the body can't be forced, we need to find ways to let relaxation happen. If our tissues aren't relaxed, supple, and pliable, they can't be rebalanced and regenerate. Getting massage therapy or taking an Epsom salt bath can be very useful for relaxing the body and removing tension from the equation.

You may also want to try mindful breathing—a kind of meditation practice where you relax your body and pay close attention to the rhythm and flow of your breath. Simple as it is, focusing on the simple act of breathing in an intentional way can help to reduce stress and tension on the body.

A MINDFUL BREATHING PRACTICE

Start by breathing in through your nose, paying close attention to the feeling of your stomach rising and your ribs separating on the inhale. Imagine a circle around your ribs from front to back, and try to expand your rib cage outward, 360 degrees, as you inhale to enlarge the circle as much as possible. Breathe slowly out through your mouth, paying attention to the feeling of your abdomen moving toward your spine and your ribs moving closer together, as you make the circle as small as you can. Repeat three times.

Whether we're conscious of it or not, we are constantly tensing our muscles and fascia. Our muscles work in teams; when one muscle is not functioning well, another compensates. This compensation can lead to the muscle working overtime and tensing up. In another instance, when a joint is inflamed, we involuntarily tense the muscles in the surrounding area to protect it. If we're feeling angry or anxious, we respond by tensing the muscles in our neck, back, and shoulders. A little attention to relaxing our emotional state when we are in pain can go a long way.

A PRACTICE FOR REDUCING TENSION

Releasing tension trapped in the muscles and fascia can help us heal, so it's useful to become more aware of your own muscular tension—how much you're carrying in a given moment and how easily you can let it go. Let's try an experiment: Ball up your hand into a fist and clench it as hard as you can for 30 seconds. Observe the sensations in your hand as you clench it tighter. How does your palm feel? Your thumb and fingers? Let go. Observe the sensations as you relax, breathe out, and release the tension. Notice how it feels as your muscle cells flood with oxygen, dissipating the tension even further.

Try doing a mindful body scan, breathing and relaxing every muscle in your body one at a time, starting with your left foot. First, tense the muscles in your foot as much as you possibly can while you inhale comfortably, and then relax and release all the tension as you exhale. Repeat this as you move through parts of your body.

Create a tension scale, with 10 being the most tense and 0 the most relaxed your body can feel. You can use the tension scale to assess each part of your body. As you become more aware of the physical sensations in your body, you'll learn to stop tensing your muscles when you're upset or in pain. This technique is a great tool for developing kinesthetic awareness and for listening to your muscles.

5. Learn from Your Pain

Once you get in the groove and have a great movement routine, it can be devastating to lose it, and an injury can do just that. But does it have to? I've met many people who would answer yes to this question, and I might have even said yes myself at the beginning of my career. But now I'm different. I've developed an attitude of gratitude.

I know first-hand that it can be really tough when pain sneaks up on you and you can't do what your mind thinks you should be able to do. It's disheartening if you think your body has let you down. But really, your body can only respond to what you give it. And if we don't give to our body, it simply can't give back.

At first, I wasn't quite so benevolent toward my body when I hurt. I felt betrayed. *How dare there be pain in my shoulder! I can't play tennis! I worked so hard and now I'm sidelined.* I found it really tough. I was used to being active every day, and I needed my movement fix. Being mad at our bones and joints doesn't help the healing, and in fact, it puts our energy in the wrong place. Anger and frustration create muscular tension and can actually prevent healing.

I have learned this the hard way. I was not so good at relaxing, but I adjusted. I learned from watching some of my patients who were able to accept an injury and move on. I was fascinated by how quickly some people could heal. I can't emphasize enough the important role of the mind in your recovery from an injury.

Try to develop your own unique visualization for healing. Whether you're dealing with a broken bone or a torn tendon, there will be a gap that needs to be healed. I have encouraged some of my patients to visualize a metaphor for healing, such as building a bridge, filling in potholes, or melting ice as examples of bridging gaps and releasing scar tissue. I particularly like using a construction site as my visualization metaphor. I see the first group of workers going in and removing damaged tissue, cleaning up the area in preparation for repair. Then a second crew comes to the construction site, bringing in new materials and starting the repair. You can visualize the tissue that needs to be repaired and use metaphors like building a bridge or growing a flower, whatever scenario resonates with you. You can also visualize doing what you love to do, seeing yourself in action, practising your craft. Be creative and pick a metaphor for healing that resonates with you; it can be anything, so long as you feel connected to it.

It hasn't been proven that visualizing healing works, but it will not hurt you—and one thing we *do* know is that it is a powerful tool for improving athletic performance. One study compared three groups of novice basketball players learning a free-throw shot. The first group practised the shot for one hour per day for six weeks. The second group lay on a couch and visualized throwing the shot. And the third group did neither. The group that practised the visualization performed just as well as the group that had been physically practising. Our brain doesn't seem to know the difference between visualizing doing an activity and actually performing the movement!

To enhance the potential power of visualization, feel your body doing the action, hear the sounds, and bring as many senses into the visualization as you can. Pay attention to the details. You will be pleasantly surprised how visualization transfers into your physical performance once you get back to your activity.

Efficient healing is a combination of accepting the injury and focusing on what you *can* control during the healing process. It turns out you can control a lot: applying ice, doing the necessary exercises, eating healthily, and modifying your activities. And your attitude. If you listen to your body, it will tell you when you're ready to take the next step. Thinking of it this way, healing became a rewarding experience for me. Has my pain decreased? Has my swelling diminished? Have I got a better range of motion? Each of these steps was a victory and motivated me to keep going. Pain can be an opportunity to learn more about yourself.

When you're hurting, you might even use the downtime to focus on some other part of your body, improving mobility or strength there. If you have a torn Achilles tendon and you can't run, do exercises for your hips, toes, core, or arms. Do little isometrics to keep the muscles in your foot and calf busy so that when the time comes for them to get to work, they are ready. It's like idling in the car waiting for the light to turn green. You will get through the intersection faster if your vehicle is turned on and primed. Keep your engine running while you're waiting for your injury to heal.

MOVEMENT MESSAGES

- Make movement longevity a priority. Plan for daily movement, and put it in your schedule.
- Make movement a habit. Pair your daily movement routine with something else you do every day. If you do a movement routine right after you brush your teeth in the morning, while you watch the evening news, or after you wash your face in the evening, you'll be more likely to stick with it and stay active.
- Take a moment for yourself. The gifts of mobility and movement longevity will help you maintain your health and independence.
- Connect with others while you move, and enjoy being a role model for healthy living.

CHAPTER 12

Movement Longevity Schedule

If you're not experiencing any movement-related pain in your joints or muscles, that's great news. However, unless you actively work to keep things that way, the chances are good that you will experience issues as you get older.

The Movement Longevity Schedule is designed to touch on the most common areas of dysfunction to ensure all of your muscles and joints are working like they should, preventing imbalances, compensations, pain, and injuries before they start.

To keep yourself moving freely and without pain, cycle through this schedule continuously throughout the year. Just like you change the oil of your car once or twice a year to keep the engine running smoothly and to prevent more catastrophic and expensive damage, you can perform regular maintenance on your Foundation for Movement.

Ideally you'll find 15 minutes per day to give to your body, but we all know that life happens. Choose the best option from the schedules below based on your available time and preferences. You are also free to design your own schedule. If you decide to go this route, aim to perform each routine at least six times total over a four-week period. Doing the routines frequently enough will allow your brain and body to adapt for lasting results.

Repeat the Foundation for Movement Complete Screening Test (page 211) after you have completed a cycle through a Movement Longevity Schedule. This will allow you to catch those pesky imbalances before they become painful injuries. If you find that you are lacking in one area, do a more intensive session in that zone. You can share these routines with a personal trainer or physical therapist, and ask them to help build upon your foundation and performance over time. And who knows, when you repeat the Complete Foundation Movement Screen, you may find significant improvements.

Whatever schedule you choose, remember to repeat it regularly to ensure your body is tuned up and ready to support you and your active life.

Schedule 1: Five Days per Week, Six-Week Cycle

If you are short on time but committed to your foundation, perform one routine five days per week for a total of six weeks. Each routine takes about 15 minutes.

Day 1	Day 2	Day 3	Day 4	Day 5
Head, Neck, and Upper Back *(page 75)*	Knees *(page 146)*	Shoulders and Arms *(page 101)*	Low Back and Hips *(page 124)*	Ankles and Feet *(page 163)*

Schedule 2: Four Days per Week, Four-Week Cycle

Designed for those who can dedicate a bit more time per session, you will perform two routines on workout days. This schedule increases the total number of times you perform each routine over a shorter period of time. Each routine takes about 15 minutes.

	Day 1	Day 2	Day 3	Day 4
Week 1	Head, Neck, and Upper Back *(page 75)* Knees *(page 146)*	Shoulders and Arms *(page 101)* Ankles and Feet *(page 163)*	Low Back and Hips *(page 124)* Head, Neck, and Upper Back	Shoulders and Arms
Week 2	Low Back and Hips Ankles and Feet	Head, Neck, and Upper Back Knees	Shoulders and Arms Ankles and Feet	Low Back and Hips Head, Neck, and Upper Back
Week 3	Knees Shoulders and Arms	Low Back and Hips Ankles and Feet	Head, Neck, and Upper Back Knees	Shoulders and Arms Ankles and Feet
Week 4	Low Back and Hips Head, Neck, and Upper Back	Knees Shoulders and Arms	Low Back and Hips Ankles and Feet	Head, Neck, and Upper Back Knees

Schedule 3: Seven Days per Week, Six-Week Cycle

Designed for those who want to prioritize their movement health and who like the routine of a daily habit, this schedule has you focusing on one area of your body each day. Each routine takes about 15 minutes.

	Sun	Mon	Tue	Wed	Thu	Fri	Sat
Week 1	Head, Neck, and Upper Back *(page 75)*	Shoulders and Arms *(page 101)*	Low Back and Hips *(page 124)*	Knees *(page 146)*	Ankles and Feet *(page 163)*	Head, Neck, and Upper Back	Shoulders and Arms
Week 2	Low Back and Hips	Knees	Ankles and Feet	Head, Neck, and Upper Back	Shoulders and Arms	Low Back and Hips	Knees
Week 3	Ankles and Feet	Head, Neck, and Upper Back	Shoulders and Arms	Low Back and Hips	Knees	Ankles and Feet	Head, Neck, and Upper Back
Week 4	Shoulders and Arms	Low Back and Hips	Knees	Ankles and Feet	Head, Neck, and Upper Back	Shoulders and Arms	Low Back and Hips
Week 5	Knees	Ankles and Feet	Head, Neck, and Upper Back	Shoulders and Arms	Low Back and Hips	Knees	Ankles and Feet
Week 6	Head, Neck, and Upper Back	Shoulders and Arms	Low Back and Hips	Knees	Ankles and Feet	Head, Neck, and Upper Back	Shoulders and Arms

CHAPTER 13

Surgery and Other Interventions

Injuries can be overwhelming, especially if you learn that some part of your body is torn or badly damaged. Often when people hear that something is wrong (a torn meniscus or rotator cuff tendon, herniated spinal disc, etc.), they assume surgery is needed to fix it. It's a natural assumption. Something is broken, so we should fix it, and surgery seems to be the common sense solution. However, over the last 30 years, I have learned that surgery is not always the best answer, and there are other interventions you can try before going under the knife—the first of which is following the advice in this book to build new movement patterns.

Consider Surgery Carefully

I don't know how many times patients have been referred to me with "shoulder pain," and their referring doctor found evidence of a rotator cuff tear. As soon as we find something torn, we assume that it is the cause of our pain. We all want a reason or explanation for the pain. But many times, after I've looked at a patient's history and done a physical examination, it is apparent that the damaged structure on the MRI was not the cause of pain. The pain was actually coming from an adjacent muscle or from a different joint and referred to the shoulder.

For example, it is extremely common for pain to radiate from the neck to the shoulder. If I had operated on the torn rotator cuff seen on the MRI when the pain was radiating from the neck, I would not be addressing the primary cause of the pain. The person may feel better while they're recovering from surgery, but as soon as they returned to their usual activities, the pain would likely come back, because I hadn't addressed the root cause.

I believe it is important to do no harm, so rebalancing the body and sifting through the movement issues can allow the real problem area to either heal or progress and declare itself. Surgery should be a last resort. If you are not sure what is causing the pain, then you cannot be sure where to operate.

As you learned in the introduction, I have given corrective exercises to many of my patients and observed that injuries often heal when you fix why the tissues have broken down—or at least they become asymptomatic. I'm not the only one to notice this.

There has been an evolution in decision-making for surgical procedures over my professional career. For example, degenerative meniscus tears in the knee were almost always treated with surgery 30 years ago. The meniscus is a shock absorber in the knee and can degenerate and tear over time. Many times, the meniscus is the first part of the knee to wear out. If there was a torn meniscus, why not remove the tear? That should cure the patient's pain. What we have learned over the years, however, is that the meniscus damage is often a precursor to wear and tear arthritis, and removing the damaged portion of the meniscus has no advantage in preventing the development of arthritis over time. Subsequent studies compared arthroscopic surgery to rehabilitation in the treatment of meniscus tears, and the results are similar. No benefit is derived from the surgical intervention. In fact, studies now show that exercise may be superior in delaying or even preventing future surgeries on an arthritic knee.

I have always been a conservative surgeon. If I am not changing the natural history of the problem by doing surgery, or fixing a structure to improve function, what is the point of the surgery? It is crucial to understand the functional implications of the structural damage. Can we function without it? Can the damaged area become asymptomatic if we change how we use that part of the body? Our bodies have a truly amazing capacity to heal and adapt.

How do you know if the injury will heal itself or if you need to have surgery to fix the problem? Of course, you need to see a surgeon to discuss your individual case. The surgeon should address your general health, lifestyle, and overall activity demands. This helps to determine the risks associated with an anaesthetic and the potential for avoiding an operation if the symptoms could resolve and not cause further problems once the acute injury has settled. Is the tissue still partially connected? Is there a good blood supply to the area? Can we restore a Foundation for Movement without that tissue working properly? If the answer to these questions is yes, there is the potential for healing without surgery. On the other hand, if the area is very badly damaged, surgery can be needed to reattach or replace tissues. Even when surgery is a good option, it's important to restore a Foundation for Movement; it is the key to maintaining pain-free function.

A good history and physical examination combined with scans such as X-rays or MRIs can establish a diagnosis. But understanding the root cause of your pain and the natural history of the problem are essential to your recovery. Talk to your doctor and ask the right questions to help you decide if surgery is the best option. I always recommend taking a friend or family member with you for support and to write down the answers to your questions. The thought of surgery can be scary, so bring someone with you as another set of eyes, ears, and reason.

ESSENTIAL QUESTIONS TO ASK YOUR SURGEON

1. Why did my body break down?
2. Can it heal on its own without surgery?
3. What is the procedure being recommended, and how will it work?
4. Can I expect full recovery of range of motion and joint stability, and what are the benefits of the surgery?
5. Will I still have pain after the surgery? How will that be different if I don't do the surgery?
6. If I don't do surgery right away, can it still be done in a year if I don't respond to other treatments?
7. Are there alternative surgeries or treatments for my condition?
8. What will the effect of surgery be in ten years' time? Will there be any difference if I do not have the surgery?

9. Would it be worthwhile to get a second opinion?
10. What are the risks and complications of doing the surgery?

Interventions You Should Know About

If you're determined to avoid surgery for as long as possible, there are other options to manage your symptoms. It's important to know, however, that in most cases these are band-aid solutions if you don't get to the root cause and change your movement patterns. Each of the treatment variables discussed here can add some value to your recovery, but don't limit your treatment to these temporary measures. Get to the root cause of your wear and tear issue so that these band-aids don't fall off.

ICE AND HEAT

Is there swelling around the joint or muscle? Ice it. Is the tendon and/or joint stiff? Heat it. Apply the ice or heat for 15 minutes each. That said, people's bodies are different. Some of my patients do not feel good if they apply ice or heat. Try ice or heat as outlined above, maybe start with five minutes, and see how you feel. If your body does not like it—as in, it remains stiff and swollen—switch it up and substitute ice for heat or vice versa.

BRACES

There are two types of braces for wear and tear injuries: rehab braces and functional braces. Rehab braces help protect and secure a joint during recovery and are generally temporary. Functional braces support the normal function of the joint. For example, if you've torn your medial collateral ligament (MCL), you'll probably be custom-fitted with a brace to keep the joint aligned when performing strenuous activity. The custom brace holds your leg and restrains the knee's range of motion so it won't give way. Some people use braces instead of having surgery to repair a ligament.

Braces also help to provide sensory feedback about where your body is positioned in space, as they apply pressure to the skin. This helps our neuromuscular system function optimally.

KINESIOLOGY TAPE

If you've watched any track and field events in the last few years, I'm sure you've seen it: that neon-coloured tape criss-crossing players' muscles. While the marketing for kinesiology tape is often couched in complicated language, the premise behind it is simple: If placed correctly, the tape helps protect injured soft tissues by shifting the tension elsewhere and activating healthy muscles. However, like all tape, kinesiology tape easily loses its structural integrity, especially over the course of an intense activity.

For a similar but much more effective treatment, I recommend a compression wrap made by 2XU or Bauerfeind. Unlike kinesiology tape, compression garments maintain their structure, even during sweaty and competitive play, and they won't make you squeal with pain every time you take them off.

THERAPY OPTIONS

You may wonder if massage, physiotherapy, or chiropractic management will help your pain. These practitioners use different modalities such as laser, ultrasound, soft tissue release, and joint manipulation to manage your symptoms. And you may well feel better, noticing improved tissue quality due to decreased swelling and relaxation of tight tissues. This will naturally help to improve range of motion and decrease pain. However, the effects will only be temporary if you do not address your root movement issues and restore your Foundation for Movement. So, if you have the cash and a good therapist, get some help to speed things along, but be sure to do your foundational routine right after you see them.

CORTISONE INJECTIONS

Wear and tear injuries often cause inflammation, and excess inflammation creates a toxic environment, making an injury hard to heal. Cortisone injections reduce the inflammation, thereby making the injury easier to heal. For instance, if you're suffering from a knee injury and all the swelling and inflammation is restricting your range of motion, a cortisone injection could help bring that swelling and inflammation down, allowing you to move more freely, activate those affected muscles, and heal. An injection of cortisone is a band-aid solution. It does not get to the root movement issue, so after your injection, do foundational movements so that you fix the problem and don't need more injections. I always recommend using cortisone injections judiciously. Multiple cortisone injections can lead to ruptured tendons and atrophied tissues, and with needles, there's always the risk of infection.

BIOLOGICAL INJECTIONS

Sometimes there's simply too much wear and tear for the body to repair. In those cases, the increasingly popular biological injections—such as stem cells or platelet-rich plasma (PRP)—might do the trick. Stem-cell and PRP injections work by introducing extra growth and healing factors to direct the cells to remodel and repair. Thus far, research on the subject has been encouraging. In 2013, *Arthroscopy: The Journal of Arthroscopic & Related Surgery* reported that stem-cell injections were "effective for reducing pain and improving knee function in patients being treated for knee osteoarthritis," adding that stem cells had "great potential as therapeutic agents in regenerative medicine because of their multilineage potential, immunosuppressive activities, limited immunogenicity and relative ease of growth in culture." These injections do not get to the root cause of your movement dysfunction, so you need to change how you move in addition to having the injection. I personally only recommend these injections if you have tried the foundational corrections and find that the structure is too badly damaged to heal on its own. Speciality clinics offer these injections more commonly these days, but they are expensive and will not fix why you broke. Make sure you also invest in your body with exercise if you go this route.

SYNVISC INJECTIONS

Synvisc is a brand-name injection to treat arthritis that, in the words of the manufacturer, "supplements the fluid in your knee to help lubricate and cushion the joint." The idea behind Synvisc, and its competitors, is to use a fluid called hyaluronic acid, which occurs naturally in the body, to reduce inflammation and restore the knee's natural function.

If you have pain and swelling in a joint without any serious mechanical problems (think clicking, locking, or instability), a Synvisc injection will probably help. However, if you do have a serious mechanical issue with your knee, you need to address that first. And as with all injections, there's a risk of infection, however slight. Use them judiciously.

And as with all these modalities, you need to establish your Foundation for Movement as well as having the injection.

MOVEMENT MESSAGES

- MRI abnormalities are common, affecting more than 50 percent of the population over age 50. Correlate the findings with the symptoms to make an accurate diagnosis.
- Pathology identified on an MRI doesn't automatically mean you need surgery.
- Weigh the risks and benefits of surgery to fix a structure and improve your function.
- Fixing the underlying movement problems prior to surgery will clarify the issue; you may even heal and get better without surgery. Even if you don't, you will get a better result after surgery.
- Common treatments beyond surgery include modalities such as applying ice or heat, massage therapy, and injections. All will help with your symptoms but not fix the underlying cause of your body breakdown. Do the Foundation for Movement Complete Screening Test and do your recommended exercises alongside these band-aid interventions.

CONCLUSION

Don't Stop Moving

Thank you for sharing your movement journey with me. I hope this is just the beginning, and you are inspired to deepen your relationship with your body. Giving our bodies a little attention every day works wonders. They really are magic. It never ceases to amaze me the tremendous healing capacity that we can unleash so long as we give our tissues what they need.

In this book, I have focused on the physical aspects of movement and how they can direct the remodelling and healing processes of our musculoskeletal tissues in relation to wear and tear injuries. Understanding what a Foundation for Movement is, and how to maintain it, will only increase your movement longevity and quality of life.

Life is a continuous cycle of stressful encounters, and we need enough physical stress to keep us alive and thriving but not so much that we break. Accumulated over time, the little everyday stresses can lead to our foundation dissolving if we don't observe ourselves, listen to our bodies, and exercise mindfully. A little time spent every day giving to your body will allow you to stay in the regeneration phase of life. Remember you don't ever want to stop moving; just change *how* you move to give your musculoskeletal system the best chance of staying balanced.

Who is "listening" to your body? Is it your mind, your soul, or something else? Expanding your horizons to survey the emotional, nutritional, and even spiritual aspects of healing can only enhance your physical healing and therefore your movement. Considering what you eat and what you think will grow your movement repertoire and balance. I have always been amazed at the difference in healing between two patients with the same pathology but different approaches to life.

I have observed that this often comes down to a simple approach of giving the physical body the food, water, time, and emotional support that it needs to heal. Getting out of the body's way and letting it do its own thing can produce miracles. The body has an inherent intelligence. I encourage you to explore the nutritional aspects of healing to create an anti-inflammatory environment for your body.

But the power of the mind is not to be overlooked. I urge you to spend some mindful minutes reflecting on your physical body and how much you love and appreciate your muscles, bones, and joints and all they do for you. It might sound more superstitious than scientific—and everyone has their own perspective—but I believe what's happening in our minds has a profound effect on our bodies. One thing is for sure: At every level of our being something is moving. From the atomic to the molecular to the cellular up to the whole organism, things are moving. In this book, I have shared what I know about keeping everything in motion, including my secrets for maintaining a Foundation for Movement, which I believe is the key to movement longevity. What it all comes down to is this: Use it or lose it. Don't stop moving; just change how you move.

Foundation for Movement Complete Screening Test

Use the screening tests below to determine which key areas of your body to focus on when building your Foundation for Movement.

Head, Neck, and Upper Back

DO YOU HAVE FORWARD HEAD POSTURE?

1. Stand up straight with your back against the wall with your heels, buttocks, and shoulders touching the wall. There should be a small space between the wall and your lower back. Tuck your chin and see if you can touch the back of your head to the wall. Keep your eyes looking straight ahead. If you have to tilt your chin up or you cannot touch the back of your head to the wall, you likely have forward head posture.

2. The other way to measure this is to take a picture of yourself from the side while standing naturally. Make sure that your shoulder, hip, and knees are aligned. Once you have the picture, draw a line from the middle of your ear straight down. This line should meet the centre of your shoulder. If the line from your ear sits in front of your shoulder, you have forward head posture.

To resolve forward head posture, do the Head, Neck, and Upper Back Routine (page 75).

Shoulders and Arms

DO YOU LACK A STRONG FOUNDATION IN YOUR SHOULDERS?

1. Standing up straight, reach one arm up and over your head, while resting your opposite hand by your side. Turn your palm to face your back, and reach down between your shoulder blades as far as you can. Hold this position. Using your opposite hand with your palm facing out, reach for your other hand from below. Try to touch your hands together. If you can touch, you pass the test, which means your shoulder foundation is solid. If not, ask a buddy to measure the distance between your fingers. This will give you a benchmark so you can measure your progress after doing the exercises below. Those with hypermobility (super flexible joints) should be mindful not to stick out their chest and abdomen to make their hands connect. For the best assessment, your chest and abdomen should remain in a neutral position.

2. Repeat the test, raising the opposite arm overhead. It is very common to fail this test when your dominant side is reaching from below. The goal is to be able to touch your fingers to one another regardless of which arm is overhead, or at least decrease the distance between them over time.

If you lack a foundation in your shoulders, do the Shoulder and Arm Routine (page 101).

Low Back and Hips

DO YOU HAVE A TIGHT HIP POCKET AND/OR SPINE DEFICIENCIES?

1. Lie on the floor with your legs stretched out straight.

2. Use your hands to pull one of your knees up toward your chest. Observe if you can touch your knee to your chest without the opposite thigh coming off the floor.

3. Can you bring your hip up past a 90-degree angle? If you can flex your hip beyond 90 degrees, when doing so does your knee point to your armpit or to the outside of your shoulder?

4. Test the opposite leg.

If you cannot flex your hip beyond 90 degrees, the resting leg comes up off the floor, or your knee points to the outside of your shoulder, do the Low Back and Hip Routine (page 124).

DO YOU HAVE A WEAK CORE OR LOW ENDURANCE?

1. Lie on one side with your shoulders, hips, and legs in a straight line. Stagger your feet, so your top foot is in front of the bottom and both lie on the floor.
2. Position your forearm closest to the ground perpendicular to your shoulder.
3. Lift yourself off the ground with your forearm into a side plank and hold for 30 seconds.
4. Test the opposite side.

If you cannot hold yourself off the ground for 30 seconds, follow the Low Back and Hip Routine (page 124) to improve your core strength.

Knees

DO YOU HAVE TIGHT QUADRICEPS AND HIP MUSCLES?

1. Find a firm surface where you can safely lie back and hug both knees to your chest with your buttock positioned just at the surface's edge. This could be your bed, the top of a staircase, a sturdy dining room table, or the stretching table at your local gym. With your buttock at the edge of the surface, release one leg at a time and let gravity pull it toward the ground. If your hip extends so that your leg is parallel to the surface, your psoas is not tight. If your knee does not naturally hang at a 90-degree angle and remains somewhat extended, your quads are tight. Finally, if your leg pops off to the side, the muscle at the side of your hip, the iliotibial (IT) band, is tight.
2. To determine if you are not using your gluteal muscles properly and are quadriceps dominant, take a picture of yourself from the side while standing naturally. Draw a line straight up from your ankle (centred on the outside ankle bone or fibula). Your hip, shoulder, and ear should line up

perfectly with one another. If your hips sit in front of the line, you are quadriceps dominant.

If any of these muscles are tight or if you are quadriceps dominant, it will affect the function of your knee and potentially cause an injury down the road. Do the Knee Routine (page 146) to release the quadriceps and hip muscles.

Ankles and Feet

DO YOU HAVE STIFF ANKLES AND SLEEPY FEET?

1. Test your ankle dorsiflexion. Start by kneeling with one knee on the ground and the opposite knee stacked directly above your ankle. Your front foot should be about a hand width away from a wall. Try to touch your front knee to the wall while keeping that foot perpendicular to the wall and its heel in contact with the ground. If you have a stiff ankle, you may try to compensate by twisting your hips, shifting your ankle off the perpendicular, or lifting your heel off the ground. Notice if you are trying to compensate. Does your knee touch the wall? If it does, congrats, you pass the ankle dorsiflexion test! This indicates good dorsiflexion for general movement. If it does not touch, you have work to do. Test both ankles.

2. Test your ability to activate the small muscles in your feet. Stand with your feet one fist width apart, your second toes facing forward. Test one foot at a time. With your weight evenly distributed across your feet, try to lift your big toe up while keeping the other four toes down. Don't let your weight shift to the big toe or little toes as you do this. Then try to keep the big toe down and lift the other four toes up. Again, hold even pressure across the foot while controlling your toe movements. If you cannot do this, do not worry; you can teach your toes to move again. Test both feet.

If you have a weak foundation in your ankles and feet, do the Ankle and Foot Routine (page 163).

How to Recover from Injury

There are two main reasons people suffer from wear and tear pain:

1. They have no Foundation for Movement.
2. They attempt to perform an activity that is higher up the Performance Pyramid than their current physical abilities will allow.

Phase 1: Re-establish Your Foundation

IMPROVE TISSUE QUALITY

Allow the tissues to heal and improve tissue pliability by decreasing inflammation and fibrosis by using a combination of ice/heat and active self-myofascial release (ASMR), followed by isometric contractions. Practise mindful breathing (page 192), use a practice for reducing tension (page 193), and visualize healing (page 194).

RESTORE ALIGNMENT TO YOUR BODY

ASMR and isometric contractions can also help restore normal alignment and joint centration. Perform your exercises in front of a mirror so that you are aware of your body alignment.

ACTIVATE THE CORRECT MUSCLES

Re-establish proper movement patterns by using the dissociation techniques presented in the exercise routines throughout the book. Develop the proper neuromuscular movement patterns, which will correct the root movement dysfunction and protect the regenerating tissues.

RESTORE END-RANGE MOVEMENT

Actively contract the proper muscles at the limit of your range of motion to better protect your joints. Improved muscle strength throughout a controlled and expanded range of motion is the goal.

Phase 2: Move Up the Performance Pyramid

Move up the Performance Pyramid incrementally, building endurance in your reprogrammed functional movements first, followed by strength, then power, and speed—all while maintaining good technique.

The basic principles for progressing up the Performance Pyramid are:

1. Warm up using a combination of ASMR, dissociation, and ERE techniques. If you feel great, cycle through the routines in the book to keep your body fresh. If you have an area of concern, use the specific routine as recommended in the book for your warm-up.
2. Maintain good form when doing your exercise routines and your daily activities.
3. Focus on the rhythm of the action with low-intensity movements. Before returning to more intense activities or to specific motions, start by shadowing the movement without any equipment to be sure your movement patterns are consolidated. For example, mimic vacuuming without the vacuum or swinging a golf club without the club in your hand.
4. As you feel better, increase the duration of movement while maintaining lower intensity and add the tools to the action, e.g., ball, vacuum, bat, rake or other object.
5. Once you have reached the desired duration of performance, begin to increase intensity of movement over the following weeks to months, increasing in a stepwise fashion as your strength, power, and speed improve.

Dealing with Roadblocks

PAIN OR SWELLING RETURN

If you develop pain or swelling at any level of the Performance Pyramid, you must return to the previous level of activity.

- If you are higher up the pyramid in the power or speed tier, return to the strength phase.
- If you have just increased duration, decrease to your previously successful effort.
- If you have just adjusted the intensity, return to your previous level of intensity where you successfully maintained form in a pain-free manner. Stay at this level until you are pain free and your range of motion and movement pattern have improved.

LOSS OF MOBILITY

Identify what might have caused the loss. Have you have lost range of motion? Has an old movement pattern returned? Correct either of these issues with the appropriate combination of ASMR, dissociation, and ERE techniques. Retake the Foundation for Movement Complete Screening Test (page 211) to determine where you have lost your foundation.

ACKNOWLEDGMENTS

Like most of you, my life has had its ups and downs. I am so grateful to all the people who have been a part of my life, shaping my views regarding pain and thus the contents of this book. I would particularly like to acknowledge the thousands of patients over the years who have come to me in pain and shared their life stories. It has been a privilege to work with you, problem-solving and participating in your healing journey. You have taught me so much about the mind, body, and soul and how they can all come together to manifest a remarkable healing state. To witness the amazing transformation of our body and its ability to heal when given the right set of conditions has truly been a gift.

I have been writing this book for over a decade. I ran into various roadblocks along the way, mainly time constraints that prevented me from getting it all together. The good thing about the delay is that the content has evolved as I have learned even more in the past few years, which is reflected in this book. I would like to thank Colin Fleming for his initial writing and work with me to organize my thoughts and get an excellent first draft on paper. Colin, you are super smart, funny, and kind. I hope you get to share your own story in a book one day. Thank you to Doug McGinnis and his team for editing an initial draft of the book; you helped to get the language into layperson's terms. Thank you to Eric Wong for his input on some of the exercise routines. A big thank you to Marla Shoom for sharing her gym for us to take our exercise photographs, to Lisa Robertson, our photographer extraordinaire, and to Mark Shoom and Jade Robinson for demonstrating the exercises. I was going to self-publish this book until I met Steven Stein, a fellow tennis friend who encouraged me to meet with his agent, Michael Levine. Thank you to Steven for the introduction to Michael Levine, another amazing man. Michael, thank you for believing in me and constructing the publishing deal with Penguin Canada. Your experience and wisdom will help launch this book into the stratosphere. I hope this is the first of many projects together!

To my team at Penguin Canada: I must express my greatest gratitude to Laura Dosky, Justin Stoller, Alanna McMullen, Talia Abramson, and Crissy Boylan. Your endless patience and feedback have been invaluable. I must give Laura a special shout-out. Laura, your grasp of the concepts, ability to organize ideas, and strengthen the general flow of information have made this a better book. Thank you! I really enjoyed collaborating with you and working through the challenges of converting the language of a scientifically minded surgeon into user-friendly words that all can appreciate and learn from. It was really fun to try some new ideas and concepts. Some worked, and some did not, but the trial and error have resulted in a book that I am so proud of. Getting me to delete "quarterbacks" and "fascial clothing" was a task, and one that you handled with grace and good humour. I hope to work with you again!

A final thank you to my children, Hannah and Joshua, for your patience with me as a working mom. Thirty years ago, after you were born, someone asked me if I was going to go back to work! I was shocked. I had just spent 16 years honing my craft and was in my first year of practice as an orthopaedic surgeon scientist when you came along. There was no way I was going to stop working. I love what I do, *and* I love being a mom. It was not always easy to juggle all of our needs as a family unit, but I think we have done all right. Part of the reason it has taken me so long to finish this book is I had to learn how to juggle! I am so excited and proud to finally have this book on the shelf and could not be more proud of the two of you.

SELECTED REFERENCES

Agur, A. M. R., Anne M. R. Agur, and Arthur F. Dalley, eds. *Grant's Atlas of Anatomy*. 11th ed. Lippincott Williams & Wilkins, 2005.

Berg, Bjørnar, Ewa M. Roos, Martin Englund, et al. "Arthroscopic Partial Meniscectomy Versus Exercise Therapy for Degenerative Meniscal Tears: 10-Year Follow-Up of the OMEX Randomized Controlled Trial." *British Journal of Sports Medicine* 59, no. 2 (January 2025): 91–98. doi.org/10.1136/bjsports-2024-108644.

Englund, Martin, Ali Guermazi, Daniel Gale, et al. "Incidental Meniscal Findings on Knee MRI in Middle-Aged and Elderly Persons." *New England Journal of Medicine* 359, no. 11 (September 11, 2008): 1108–15. doi.org/10.1056/NEJMoa0800777.

Ham, Arthur W. *Ham's Histology*. 9th ed. Lippincott, 1987.

Jensen, M. C., M. N. Brant-Zawadzki, N. Obuchowski, M. T. Modic, D. Malkasian, and J. S. Ross. "Magnetic Resonance Imaging of the Lumbar Spine in People Without Back Pain." *New England Journal of Medicine* 331, no. 2 (July 14, 1994): 69–73. doi.org/10.1056/NEJM199407143310201.

Koh, Yong-Gon, Seung-Bae Jo, Oh-Ryong Kwon, et al. "Mesenchymal Stem Cell Injections Improve Symptoms of Knee Osteoarthritis." *Arthroscopy* 29, no. 4 (April 2013): 748–55. doi.org/10.1016/j.arthro.2012.11.017.

Maman, Eran, Craig Harris, Lawrence White, George Tomlinson, Misra Shashank, and Erin Boynton. "Natural History of Rotator Cuff Tears: Longitudinal MRI and Clinical Follow-Up of Non-operated Tears." *The Journal of Bone & Joint Surgery* 91, no. 8 (August 2009): 1898–1906. doi.org/10.2106/JBJS.G.01335.

Miniaci, A., and E. L. Boynton. "Clinical Assessment, Imaging and Classification." In *OKU Shoulder and Elbow*, edited by T. R. Norris. American Academy of Orthopaedic Surgeons, 1998.

Myers, Thomas W. *Anatomy Trains: Myofascial Meridians for Manual and Movement Therapies*. 2nd ed. Churchill Livingstone, 2009.

Sahrmann, Shirley, and associates, eds. *Movement System Impairment Syndromes of the Extremities, Cervical and Thoracic Spines*. Elsevier Mosby, 2010.

Schleip, Robert, Thomas W. Findley, Leon Chaitow, and Peter A. Huijing, eds. *Fascia: The Tensional Network of the Human Body*. Churchill Livingstone, 2012.

Sihvonen, Raine, Mika Paavola, Antti Malmivaara, et al. "Arthroscopic Partial Meniscectomy for a Degenerative Meniscus Tear: A 5 Year Follow-Up of the Placebo-Surgery Controlled FIDELITY (Finnish Degenerative Meniscus Lesion Study) Trial." *British Journal of Sports Medicine* 54, no. 22 (November 2020): 1332–9. doi.org/10.1136/bjsports-2020-102813.

Wong, Joseph Y. *A Manual of Neuro-anatomical Acupuncture Volume 1: Musculoskeletal Disorders*. The Toronto Pain and Stress Clinic Inc, 1999.

INDEX